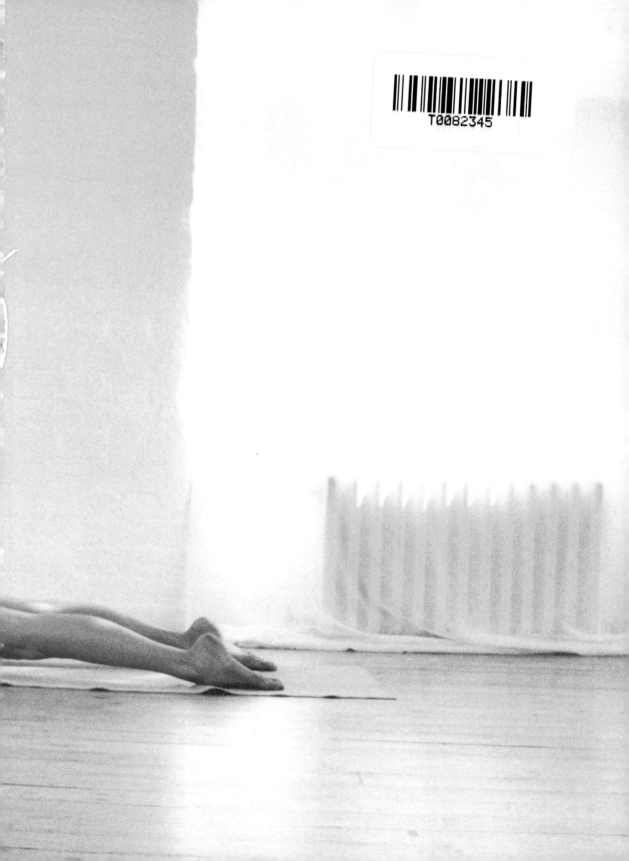

Astanga Yoga

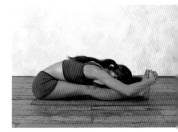

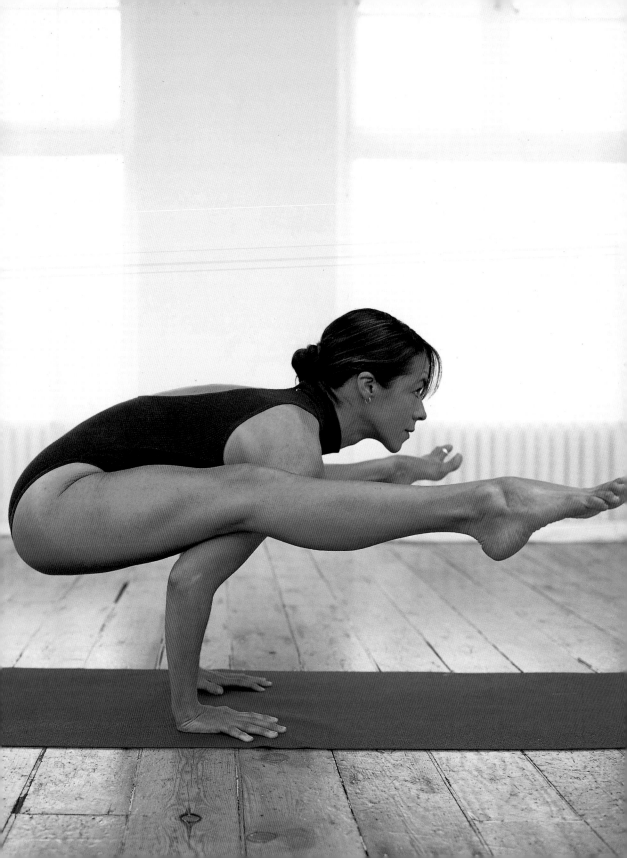

Astanga Yoga

Dynamic flowing vinyasa
yoga for strengthening
body and mind

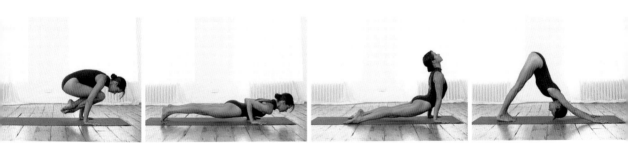

JEAN HALL

PHOTOGRAPHY BY CLARE PARK

LORENZ BOOKS

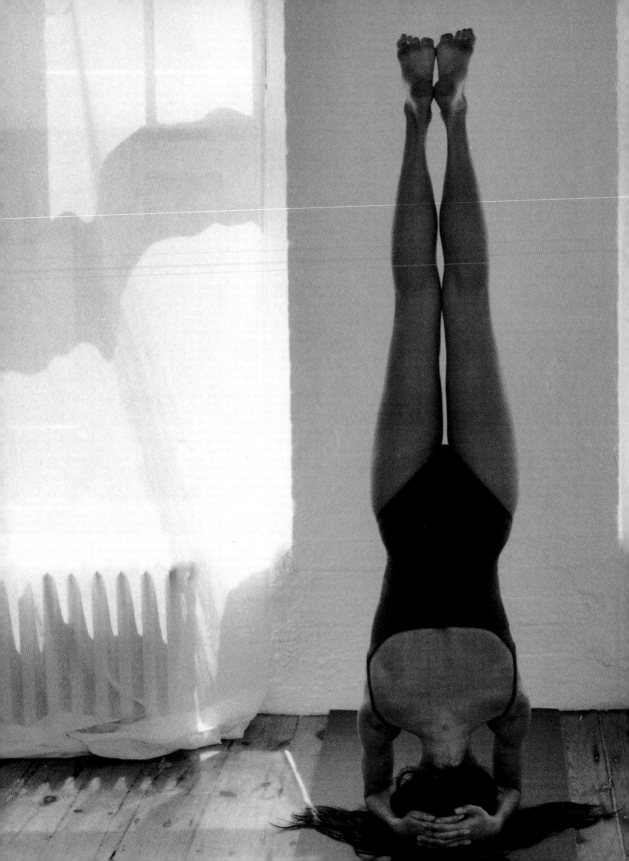

Contents

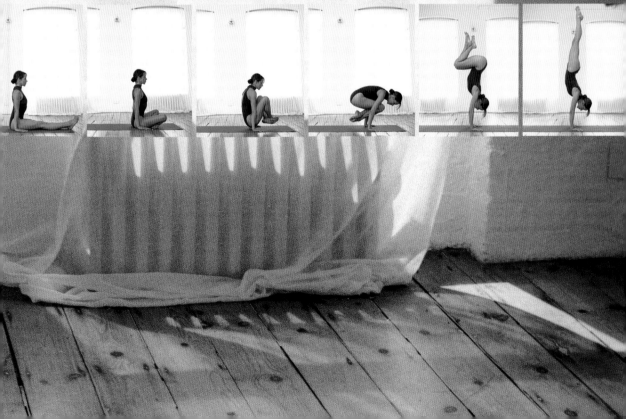

Introduction

Many centuries ago, ancient sages, mystics and diverse thinkers (also known as richies) drew upon the inspiration of life and death to reveal one of the greatest gifts to the human race: yoga.

The term "yoga" is derived from the Sanskrit language. Its meaning, "union, bringing together, connection and communion", refers to the ever-present union between the individual spirit or self, *jiva*, and the universal spirit or self, *atman*. This can also be thought of as personal consciousness connecting with global consciousness. In yogic thought, this union is considered to be real and concrete, and it is described as enlightenment or self-realization. This is the belief that none of us are separate. We are all, right now in this moment, connected – we are all one – and through the various practices of yoga we are able to realize the divine eternal spirit which connects and flows through us all.

The nature of yoga is discovered in the doing. In essence, it is a non-verbal process, an inner journey to the centre of the soul, which is the source of all happiness and ultimately self-realization of union or non-separateness.

This book is an ideal introduction to Astanga yoga for newcomers to the subject. Anyone who is already practising will find it an aid to deepening their awareness. The book begins with a short section on the background and ideas behind the exercises. The chapter on the Elements of Astanga gives you all the language and knowledge you will need in your practice. The primary series is shown in its entirety, before going into each posture in detail.

Starting our practice with a physical and sensual awakening of the body is often the first step for many of us on the yoga journey. One of the distinguishing features of Astanga yoga is the focus on the breath. It is the breath that

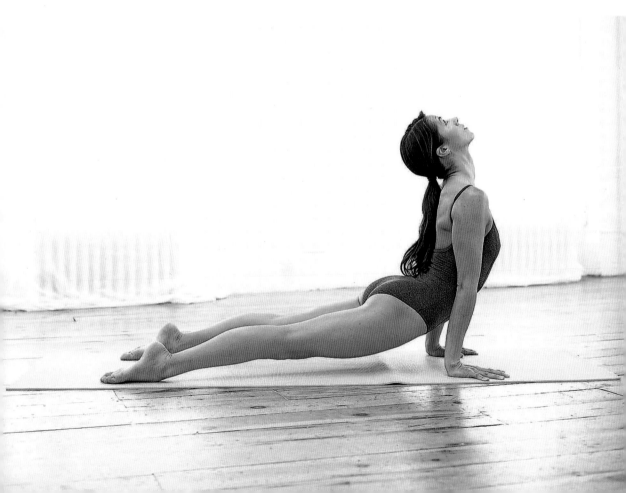

links each posture. Through the bodily practice of yoga, consciousness merges with the movement of the breath, and the body merges with the motion and stillness of the postures, or asanas. This creates physical, mental and emotional balance, openness, intelligence, strength and wellbeing, bringing body, mind and spirit into ever-greater harmony and health.

The Astanga yoga series of asanas focuses on linking the body and mind through the flowing thread of the breath. In an analogy to life, we breathe and move in and out of balance and stillness, creating an ideal situation in which we can truly feel our strengths and weaknesses, our frustrations and limitations, and can learn to be still with them and yet not get stuck with them in any one position. We keep steadily flowing – taking in and letting go with each breath.

Within this book I wish to share that which has been shared with me: the internal illumination of the personal journey that helps us to return to our own deep source and inner truth each day, connecting to the ever-profound power of the heart through the motion of the breath and body. In this way, we are able to touch all those who have gone before us, those who are present now and those who are yet to come. Thus the yogic path can lead us beyond our ordinary consciousness and personality to realize the eternal spirit of compassion and freedom.

Yoga is humanity's heritage, a living tradition of consciously realizing our completeness and oneness, through our inherent connection to all beings.

We may live the spirit of yoga – searching, exploring and evolving our practice and journey on the mat as well as in our daily lives.

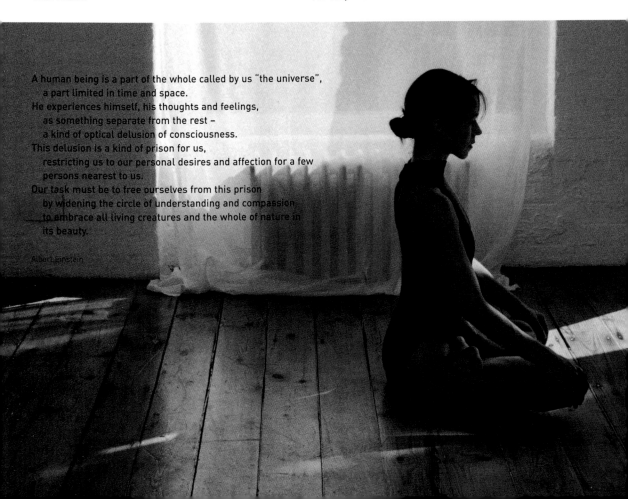

A human being is a part of the whole called by us "the universe",
    a part limited in time and space.
He experiences himself, his thoughts and feelings,
    as something separate from the rest –
    a kind of optical delusion of consciousness.
This delusion is a kind of prison for us,
    restricting us to our personal desires and affection for a few
    persons nearest to us.
Our task must be to free ourselves from this prison
    by widening the circle of understanding and compassion
    to embrace all living creatures and the whole of nature in
    its beauty.

Albert Einstein

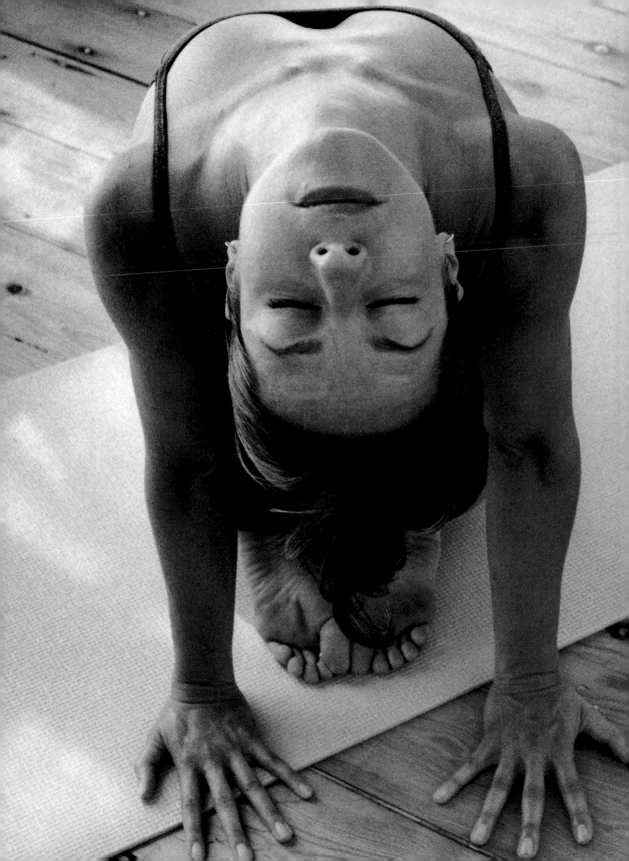

History and Philosophy

The ancient science of yoga has its seeds in the beginning of time, yet it still continues to grow and evolve. It is an alive, breathing art form, inspired from the depths of nature. It is becoming more relevant with the passage of time as it helps bring us back to our natural centre and maintain balance in our fast and ever-changing lifestyles.

In ancient times, and in original writings, the yogi was seen as someone who understood that the entire universe was present within their own body.

Astanga yoga is a form of Hatha yoga. *Hatha – ha* (sun), *tha* (moon) – is a guiding force towards the realization of universal energies within. It teaches the harnessing and integration of polar energies of the universe to create physical, mental, emotional and spiritual balance and union within.

Through the discipline of yoga postures and mental concentration, the solar aspect (yang – active, masculine) is harmonized with the lunar aspect (yin – intuitive, feminine).

Yoga's History and Philosophy

Yoga has its origins deep in pre-history and slowly evolved through the ancient Tantric civilizations that were in existence more than 10,000 years ago throughout India and in many other parts of the world. In these ancient Tantric times, the rishis (seekers and seers), finding inspiration and truth in nature, realized techniques to attain freedom from the burdens and attachments of the world while still living within it. First, recognition of the human limitations of body and mind was needed. Then methods to transcend these limitations in order to open consciousness into higher realms of reality were taught. These skills were then handed down by word of mouth from guru (teacher) to pupil throughout the generations.

Tantra, the name given to the sacred books of Tantrism, stems from *tan-oti*, meaning "expansion", and *tra-yati*, meaning "liberation". In Tantric philosophy, the body is regarded as the gateway to the inner temple of the divine. Thus the body and bodily existence was recognized on a manifest level as a wonderful instrument through which the expansion of the unmanifest consciousness (*Shiva*) and freedom of energy (*Shakti*) can be realized and united.

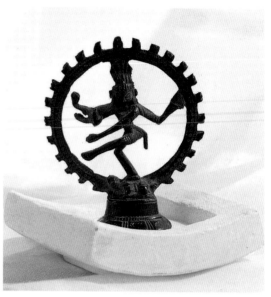

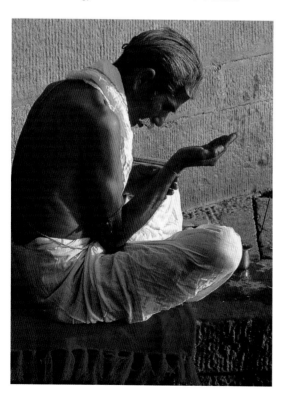

The term "yoga" emerged in written sources over 4,000 years ago in the ancient Sanskrit hymns and poems of the *Tantras* and later the *Vedas*, which refer to ritualistic traditions, folklore, esoteric practices and spiritual awakenings. These scriptures are considered to be sacred, as they were originally revealed to the rishis while they were in deep yogic states of meditation.

Further writings, called the *Upanisads* (literally meaning "to sit near the teachings"), gave clearer definition to the journey of yoga. These texts, 108 authentic books in all, are the final part of the Vedas, and the basis of Vedanta, which is one of the six philosophical systems of Indian thought. The Upanisads are diverse in their varied spiritual teachings, but in essence they reveal that the soul is at the core of us all and that therefore none of us is separate:

The Self is the Ultimate Reality
That which was before creation, And from which creation
was born
Yet who sees this Self, Sees it resting in the hearts of all.

Katha Upanisad

Above Shiva, the third god of the Hindu trinity, is here depicted in his reincarnate form of Nataraja – the Lord of Dancers. The circle of fire symbolizes the ever-turning universe in its state of eternal flux.
Left Here, a Hindu Brahmin at the bank of the Ganges performs a ritual worship known as puja. Hindus regard the river Ganges as the most sacred river in India.

This knowledge is realized not through speculation and theory but through duty, inner contemplation and meditation. The Upanisads provide the source of Astanga yoga, but they are more inspirational than instructional, with profound suppositions and revelations, both practical and poetic.

At this point in yoga's history (the Upanisads were written between 400 and 200BC), the instructional methods of yoga were still imparted personally from the guru directly to his pupil. Different teachers taught different techniques and aspects, making its development somewhat random. It was not until the great rishi Patanjali (c. 2nd century BC) systematized and compiled the existing yoga practices that had been handed down to him, along with knowledge contained in the Veda and Upanisads, that yoga was given a comprehensive format and philosophical shape. Patanjali's Yoga Sutra, meaning "yoga thread", creates the essential foundations of yoga as we know it today and is considered one of the most significant texts on yoga. Within the 196 aphorisms contained in this book, Patanjali provides the aspiring yogi with a profound structure of eight steps, or limbs (asta means "eight", anga means "limb"), to follow, like a thread, along the yogic pathway in order to reach liberation and enlightenment.

THE EIGHT LIMBS OF ASTANGA YOGA
1 **The 5 yamas** (Restraints to create inner integrity)
Ahimsa: non-violence and non-harming in any form to any living creature. This creates compassionate living, as true non-violence is a state of mind and heart.
Satya: truthfulness in mind, word and action. This is considered to be the highest law of morality.
Asteya: non-stealing, to free ourselves from possessiveness and envy.
Brahmacharya: abstinence and the practice of moderation in all things.
Aparigraha: non-greed in order to simplify life by adopting an attitude of generosity and non-hoarding.

2 **The 5 niyamas** (Ethical and moral observations)
Saucha: purity and cleanliness of mind, body, heart and environment.
Santosha: cultivation of inner contentment, in order not to hold others responsible for our happiness.
Tapas: to glow and be illuminated with an inner aim and direction in life for growth. The great yogi Iyengar suggests that a "life without Tapas is like a heart without love".
Svadhyaya: study, not only of an intellectual kind but also of oneself, to develop self-understanding of our inner nature.
Isvara-pranidhana: realization, devotion and dedication to the divine presence within all life.

3 **Asanas** (Postures)
Asana means "seat" and refers to the art of body postures that have evolved over many centuries. Apart from cultivating kanti (physical beauty) due to the enhanced pranic flow (life energy) through the body, asanas remove fickleness of mind to restore mental and physical health, strength, wellbeing and vitality. Asana practice also reflects the tendencies, strengths, weaknesses and actions in our life.

4 **Pranayama** (Breath regulation)
Prana is the vital life energy within the breath, and so it can also be translated as "the breath of life". Ayama means "expansion" or "to stretch", and therefore pranayama is the practice whereby life energy is expanded through the regulation and control of the breath. The natural sound of the breath Soham (soh-hum), in Sanskrit means "I am that... beyond the limitations of body and mind" and resonates unconsciously through the body like a mantra (sacred prayer) with each breath taken. In yoga it is believed that by listening into our breath we also become aware of this quiet blessing.

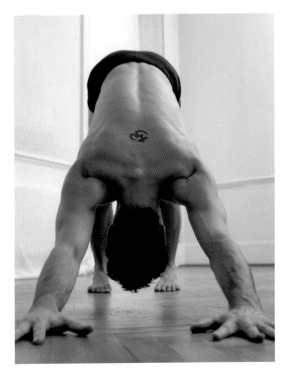

Above Adho Mukha Svanasana. Standing asanas tone the body and help to develop strength, stamina and concentration.

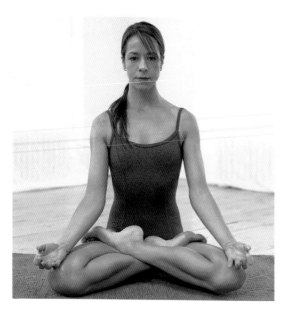

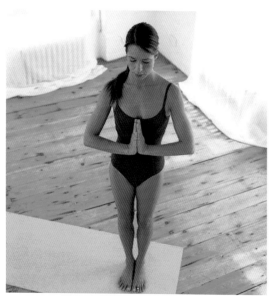

Top Sitting in Padmasana (lotus pose) with the hands in the *chin mudra* position is a comfortable and traditional way to practise meditation, focusing the mind and calming the brain (see pages 24–5).
Bottom The Mantras are recited at the beginning of one's yoga practice. This is traditionally done standing in Tadasana with the hands in Namaste, palms together as if in prayer (see page 32).

5 **Pratyahara** (Sensory withdrawal)
The ancient scriptures suggest that the entire cosmos is situated within the human body, and therefore it is understood that the source of happiness lies within each individual. By withdrawing our senses from external stimulation, we are able to connect to this inner well of contentment, rather than relying on outward sensory stimulus and grasping in order to fulfil our unquenchable desires. The process of introspection and pratyahara, which certain asanas, such as Kurmasana (tortoise posture), induce, also leads to self-understanding and acceptance.

6 **Dharana** (Concentration)
The practice of dharana, or concentration, can take many forms. Methods include being completely attentive to the flow of the breath in harmony with the movement of the body, or focusing on the glow of a candle flame, watching its movements and sharing its light. Whatever technique is used, the aim is the same – to strengthen the mind and gather psychic energies in order to move into a meditative state.

7 **Dhyana** (Meditation)
Through the practice of one directional flow of the mind, *ekatanata*, of concentration, meditation will begin to follow naturally if time is given to it. Meditation is absolute, it is where we can go beyond time, space, conditions and limitations, allowing our individual core of consciousness to expand and connect with the infinite universal consciousness. The ancient sages described meditation as yoking with nature, as they conceived the infinite universe to be part of the nature of life, death and beyond.

8 **Samadhi** (Enlightenment, bliss state of oneness)
This is the ultimate yoga, and it is the culmination of the previous seven limbs. Samadhi transcends meditation: it is without seed, as it goes beyond beginning and end; it is a state of absolute liberation and bliss in which nothing is needed, desired or required as the self has merged all.

To truly practise Astanga yoga we need to endeavour to incorporate all eight limbs: to practise the physical aspects, which are the asanas and pranayama, and to strive to live the actions of yoga, yama, niyama, pratyahara, dharana and dhyana. By reading and discussing, the concepts of yoga may be intellectually understood, but that understanding needs to be put into practice if we wish to experience the richness of its benefits and bring meaning into our lives. As Sri K. Pattabhi Jois expounded, yoga is 99 per cent practice and 1 per cent theory. This requires practice of all the eight limbs of yoga, not just the asanas.

SRI T. KRISHNAMACHARYA, SRI K. PATTABHI JOIS AND THE YOGA KORUNTA

Sri T. Krishnamacharya, one of the most influential yogis of recent times, is said to have rediscovered a lost and forgotten manuscript sitting in the recesses of the national library of Calcutta during the early 1930s. The story of this manuscript, the Yoga Korunta, may be myth or real, but it has inspired thousands of yoga practitioners from all over the world to practise yoga asana with love and devotion.

It is claimed that Sri T. Krishnamacharya together with his disciple Sri K. Pattabhi Jois, collated and deciphered this Sanskrit manuscript that was written on leaves and was barely intact when found. It is no longer in existence today but was believed to have dated back some 1,000–1,500 years.

In the Yoga Korunta a system of Hatha yoga that was created and practised by its author, a seer called Vamana Rishi, is described. The manuscript comprises hundreds of stanzas and advocates the way of the breath to integrate the eight limbs of Patanjali's Yoga Sutra. In full detail, movement and breath are described as the means into and out of the postures, with counted breaths while in each asana, advising "Oh yogi, do not do asana without vinyasa." Vinyasa means "breath-synchronized movement". It is the practice of moving the body in harmony with the breath to help induce a state of deep concentration.

Within the Yoga Korunta, three series of yoga sequences are imparted:

1 Yoga Chikitsa – yoga therapy, to align and detoxify the body and mind. This is the primary series.
2 Nadi Sodhana – channel cleansing, to purify the subtle body and energy within. This is the intermediate series.
3 Sthira Bhaga – divine stability, to create profound openness, humility and stability.

This series came to be divided into four subseries due to its demanding nature. Only when the first series has been fully understood and achieved is the next one introduced. This is the system of Hatha yoga that was taught by *Sri K. Pattabhi Jois (who died in 2009) and his grandson Sharath at the Asthanga Yoga Research Institute in Mysore, India, and since throughout the world.

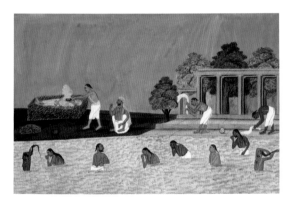

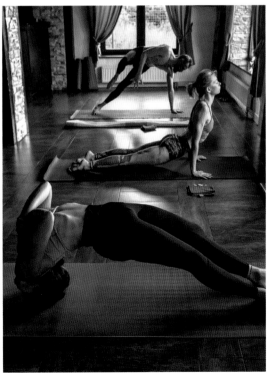

Above This painting from Trichinopoly, India, depicts *varuna snana* – or watery bathing – a component of *niyama*, to cleanse and purify the yogi's body. Bathing in sacred water, ashes, soil, sunshine, and contemplation of the divine are all forms of snana.
Right Mysore self-practice.

Footnote *Sri K Pattabhi Jois created the Ashtanga Yoga Research Institute in 1948 in Mysore where he taught this system up until his death in 2009. Since his death a substantial number of his students have revealed they were sexually abused under his tutorage. His grandson, Sharath Jois, who inherited the Ashtanga Yoga Research Institute, has publicly apologised for his grandfather's improper behaviour. Sharath nows heads the Institute and teaches with continued dedication.

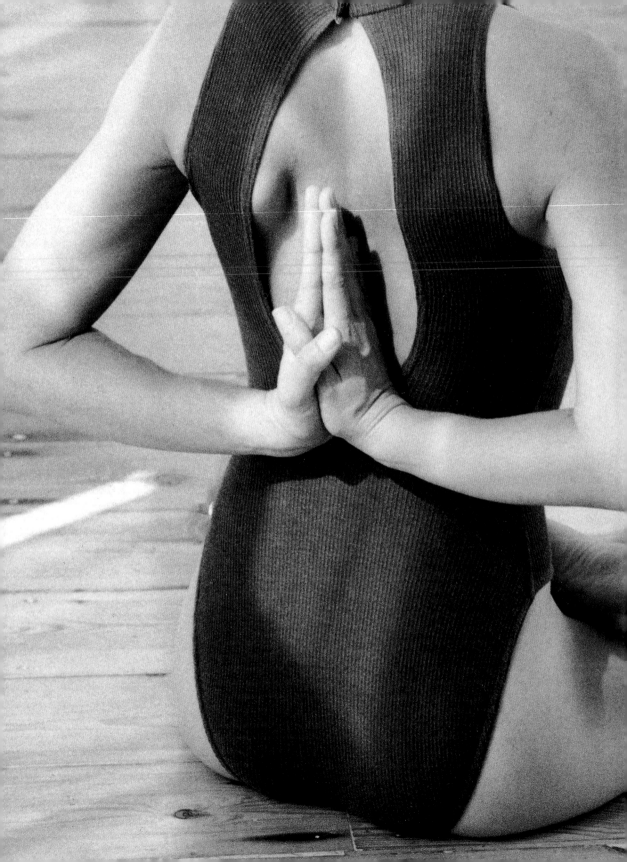

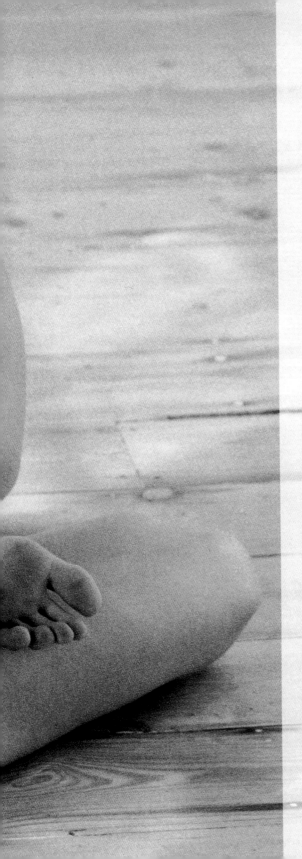

The Elements of Astanga Yoga

Astanga is a unique form of Hatha yoga that places emphasis on the flowing energy of breath, body and mind to cultivate an inner core strength. The primary instrument of Astanga yoga is the body, which is led through a sequence of yoga postures (asanas).

The distinguishing elements of Astanga yoga and its practice are weaved together with the eight limbs of Patanjali's *Yoga Sutra* to create *sadhana* – a complete spiritual practice. These elements are:
- vinyasa – breath-synchronized motion
- ujjayi pranayama – victorious breathing
- the bandhas – inner locks
- the dristis – gaze points

The outer, physical body in yoga is referred to as *Sthula-sharira* – the gross or coarse body. This cage of the physical body houses the *Sukshma-sharira* – the subtle body, which is the inner, or psychic, realm of our existence. This subtle body is not visible to the eye but is just as real as the physical, and even more powerful and profound. The subtle inner dimension of existence can be felt and experienced through deep internal awareness, pranayama and meditation.

Vinyasa

The motion of breath is the inspiration of the body and propels the body into action, and it is the essence of Astanga yoga. Vinyasa teaches us to move in harmony with the subtle and profound power of our breathing – its movement skywards with the inhalation, and its surrender earthwards on the exhalation. Vinyasa literally translates as "breath-synchronized movement", and it is the external expression of the internal motion of the breath. Through breath the life energy of prana is carried throughout the body.

Pattabhi Jois describes the system of vinyasa as a yoga *mala*. Mala means "garland" or "rosary", and in this sense, instead of a garland of flowers or rosary of prayers, vinyasa creates a garland or rosary of yoga postures, threaded together through the flow of the yoga breath. Thus each motion of the body is inspired by the motion of the breath.

The natural motion of our breathing carries our body through the practice. The breath softly lifting us up and releasing us down, motivates our body to flow in and out of the postures. This creates a continuous stream of movement in which body and mind are linked. The uniting of breath and motion symbolizes the union of the individual consciousness with the universal consciousness.

By becoming mindful of our breathing and its natural rhythm, we move into the full realms of yoga. This is because conscious linking of body, mind and breath as we move through the postures cultivates continuous concentration (dharana) on the flow of breath (pranayama) with the flow of asanas. This deep attention to the breath creates a quietening of the senses (pratyahara), preparing the pathway for the meditative state of contemplation and meditation (dhyana), which leads us towards the blissful union of the soul with the divine (samadhi). Yama and niyama can be more readily understood and absorbed as the body and mind become open and liberated through these practices.

On a physical level, vinyasa builds and maintains the heat of the body, allowing for the deep releasing stretches of the body in the asanas, while stoking the digestive fire to further the internal benefits of each posture. Another important aspect of vinyasa is that it enables us to develop our self-practice, so that we may flow at our own pace, moving to the rhythm of our own breath, drawing ourselves on every level deeper and deeper into meditation.

Vinyasa begins with Surya Namaskara; the rise and fall of the breath carries the upward and downward flow of the body from posture to posture. Through the standing asanas, we surrender into the posture with the exhalation, and move out of the posture with the inhalation. Even as we are in the stillness of each posture, the breath continues to flow, opening and releasing the body further with every breath.

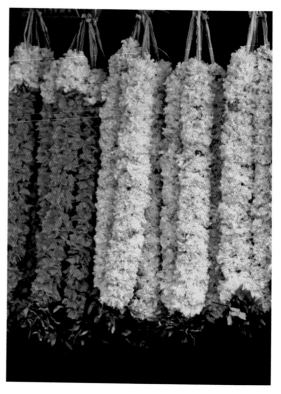

Above Yoga movements with vinyasa are described as being like a *mala*, or garland of flowers, linked together by the breath.

TO PRACTISE VINYASA

Within seated asanas, a half vinyasa is practised between each side of the posture in order to neutralize the body. After completing a sitting posture on both sides and before entering into the next new posture, a full vinyasa is practised. The full and half vinyasa sequences take their inspiration from the Surya Namaskaras, which incorporate pranayama (breath control), asanas (postures of body), dristis (focus points) and bandhas (locks or seals). It is for this reason that the flowing sequence of postures that is Surya Namaskara forms the bedrock of the physical practice of Astanga yoga.

As you flow through your practice, pay attention to the detail and alignment of each posture. Just as words are strung together to create a sentence, so the postures are linked to create the vinyasa. However, if the words are not pronounced coherently, the meaning of the sentence is lost. If the postures are not formed correctly, there will be no internal understanding, and your practice will make no sense.

Ujjayi Pranayama

Ujjayi pranayama encourages full breathing, so that oxygen and life can enter into our lungs and permeate every cell of the body. The word ujjayi is composed of two Sanskrit roots: *ji*, which means "to conquer or to be victorious", and the prefix *ud*, meaning "bondage". Thus ujjayi is the method of breathing that conquers bondage and liberates the mind. The breathing practice of ujjayi creates a soft resonating sound as the breath is drawn through the back of the throat on its way down into the lungs. This enables us to listen consciously to our breathing, and to tune into our life force and vital energy as our breathing washes in and out of our body. The sonorous sound of ujjayi breathing becomes a gentle mantra (sacred thought or prayer) on which our mind can focus, while creating a rhythm and flow for our body to follow as we move from asana to asana.

TO PRACTISE UJJAYI PRANAYAMA

Sit in any comfortable position, keeping your back straight and your spine lengthened. Now relax your body without slumping, and draw your focus downwards or allow your eyes to close completely. Bring your awareness to your breath entering and exiting through your nostrils. Allow your breathing to become deep, slow, rhythmic and calm. Now take your awareness to your throat: feel your breath softly brushing through the back of your throat on both your inhalation and exhalation.

As your concentration deepens, become aware of the four stages of each breath cycle without exaggerating any one of them. First, there is your inhalation (*puraka*), which pours into your lower body and fills all the way to the brim of your collarbones. Second, there is a moment of suspension when your inhalation is complete but the exhalation has not begun; this is called *antara kumbhaka*. Third, there is the exhalation (*rechaka*), where the breath is released from your upper body and empties down through to your lower body. Finally, there is a gentle retention (*bahya kumbhaka*), when your exhalation is complete but the inhalation has yet to begin. Be careful just to notice antara kumbhaka and bahya kumbhaka and not to accentuate either of them.

Now begin to contract the glottis gently by moving the well of your front throat in towards your back throat, so that a soft internal sonorous sound resonates from the throat to the heart on your inhalation, and from your heart to your throat on your exhalation. The sound will resemble that of a whispering breeze or the gentle breath of a sleeping baby. The resonating vibration of the breath ripples internally rather than being projected or pushed outwards.

If you have difficulty at first in creating the sound of ujjayi pranayama, practise by inhaling and exhaling through your mouth while whispering "hhaaa" at the back of your throat with each in and out breath. Continue to whisper "hhaaa" at the back of your mouth and transfer your breathing into and out of your nose. As your practice of ujjayi pranayama deepens, be aware of upward-moving energy on the inhalation and downward-moving energy on the exhalation.

Above Sit in Padmasana (lotus pose) to practise ujjayi pranayama. If this is not comfortable for you, refer to page 26 for alternatives.

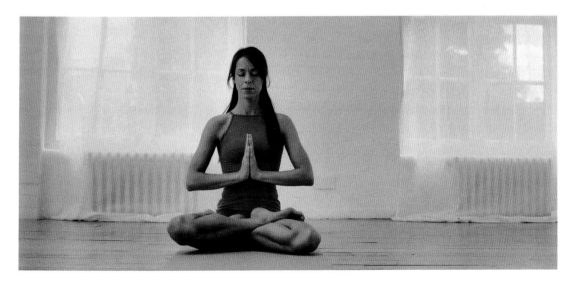

The Bandhas

The Sanskrit word bandha means "to bond, catch hold of or lock", and this is exactly the physical action involved in the creation and practice of the bandhas.

There are three primary bandhas: jalandhara bandha, uddiyana bandha and mula bandha. These bandhas, or locks, are created by gently yet powerfully contracting specific parts of the body to seal in the vital energy (prana) of the breath and redirect the pranic flow into the *sushumna nadi*, which is the subtle pathway of the spine. Once energy begins to flow through the sushumna, spiritual awakening begins.

Each bandha helps to dissipate psychic knots (called *granthis*) within the subtle body that block the free flow of prana ascending along the sushumna, thus hindering meditation and ultimately liberation. On a physical level, the bandhas form the core strength of the body and are engaged throughout the practice to provide internal support.

JALANDHARA BANDHA

The word *jala* means "a net or a mesh". This throat lock has the effect of regulating the flow of prana to the heart and the heart chakra (see page 28).

In this bandha, the front of the throat is locked by the chin being drawn down and pressed into the notch at the centre of the collarbones. In various postures, jalandhara bandha occurs naturally through the positioning of the entire body, for example in the Salamba Sarvangasana (supported whole body posture), Halasana (plough posture) and Garbha Pindasana (womb embryo posture). It may also be practised by sitting in any comfortable position, such as cross-legged or in half or full lotus (as described on pages 92 and 124).

- Place your palms down on your knees and sit with your back tall without tensing, and allow your body to relax.
- Inhale slowly and deeply.
- Draw your head forwards, lowering your chin and pressing it down firmly into the collarbone notch. Straighten your arms and press your palms securely downwards on to your knees. This will cause your shoulders to rise.
- Hold this position of jalandhara bandha for only a moment or two, then lift your chin away from your chest, release the pressure of your hands from your knees, bend your elbows and relax your shoulders down. Exhale slowly and fully. Repeat four more times.
- Throughout your asana practice, the throat lock of jalandhara bandha has its subtle form in the gentle contraction of the glottis, while ujjayi pranayama is continuously present.

Below The subtle form of uddiyana bandha strengthens the abdominal muscles, deepens the breath and, at the same time, protects the spine from injury.

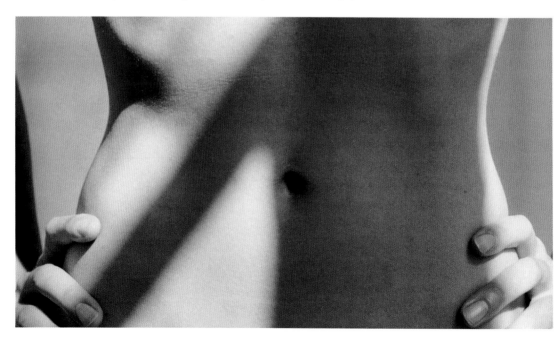

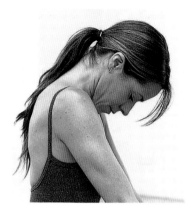

Above Jalandhara bandha

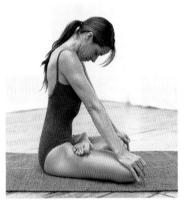

Above Uddiyana with jalandhara bandha

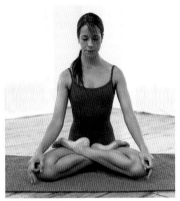

Above Mula bandha

UDDIYANA BANDHA

The word uddiyana means "to fly upwards", and it relates to the fact that the drawing in of the abdominal muscles causes the diaphragm to rise upwards. Within the subtle body, uddiyana bandha causes pranic energy to fly, like a great bird soaring upwards, along the sushumna nadi into the top chakra, thereby bringing enlightenment and ultimate union. Uddiyana bandha may be practised by sitting cross-legged, or in accomplished pose, or in half or full lotus (as described on pages 26 and 92).

- Draw your spine up straight and place your hands on your knees. Relax your body and cast your gaze downwards or close your eyes to internalize your focus.
- Breathe in slowly and deeply through your nostrils.
- Now strongly exhale through your mouth, whooshing your breath out to empty your lungs completely.
- Retain the exhalation and scoop your stomach in, contracting your abdominal muscles inwards and upwards while locking your chin down on to your collarbone notch (jalandhara bandha). Allow your shoulders to rise slightly as you firmly straighten your arms by pressing your palms down on to your knees. Do not strain and only hold for as long as is comfortable.
- To release uddiyana bandha, relax your abdomen, bend your elbows, softening your shoulders down, lift your chin and inhale slowly and gently. Let your breathing return to normal before practising uddiyana again.

The above exercise is the full expression of uddiyana bandha. However, during your asana practice it will not be possible to engage this lock to such an extreme, as it would constrict your breathing. A subtler lift upwards and inwards of the abdomen as you practise will enhance your breathing, helping you to draw your breath deeply into your back and side ribs rather than into your stomach. This will improve your lung capacity and strengthen your entire body. Be careful not to become tense as you engage uddiyana bandha. Let your abdominal muscles softly curve inwards as your breath flows into your back.

MULA BANDHA

The word mula means "root, cause or source". The location of mula bandha is at the perineal muscle, which is the muscle of the perineum area between the anus and genitals. For women, however, the contraction of this region goes deeper, so that mula bandha can be located at the cervix.

- Sit in a comfortable position (in Sukhasana, accomplished pose, or in half or full lotus).
- Lengthen your spine and relax your shoulders.
- Lower your focus or close your eyes completely and draw your awareness to the natural flow of your breath.
- Continue to breathe steadily, and take your attention to your perineal muscle or cervix. Contract this area by drawing the perineum or cervix upwards. Then relax the area. Repeat the contraction another four to five times, increasing the duration of each contraction in order to develop your strength to sustain mula bandha while breathing fully.

At first you may find you contract the anal and urinary sphincters, but with practice you will be able to refine the action of contraction into the specific area of the perineal muscle or cervix. As you practise, also be careful not to clench or grip your buttocks.

Mula bandha directs prana from the lower pelvic region upwards, helping to energize the entire body and relieve sexual frustration, guilt and suppression.

The Dristis

Our gaze point, known in Sanskrit as *dristi*, plays an important role in our practice on four different levels: practical, physical, mental and spiritual.

Of all our senses, sight and hearing are the two most compelling, continuously distracting us and drawing our mind outwards. Through our eyes we view the world outside ourselves, but we can also turn our focus inwards towards our inner life and gain insight to our true nature. As we direct our focus outwards through our open eyes, the steady vision of the dristi is a method of introspection. The outward focus is reflected inwards, focusing clearly, intently and softly, so that our open eyes are not aware of the outside world beyond our dristi.

There are nine points of focus, and each one completes the positioning of the body in each asana. The nine dristis are:

Bhru madhya: the space between the eyebrows (third eye centre, may be referred to as the *ajna chakra* or *sambhavi mudra*)
Nasagrai: the nose tip (also referred to as *agochari mudra*)
Nabi chakra: the navel
Padhayoragrai: the toes
Angustha ma dyai: the thumbs
Hastagrai: the hand
Parsva: to the right side
Parsva: to the left side
Urdhva: upwards and skywards

The prescribed dristis allow our eyes to rest on one point, helping to prevent our mental focus from being distracted during yoga practice by other visual stimulations and their associations. This helps us to develop one-pointedness – where the focus is concentrated on one single point. With practice this induces higher states of concentration that promote mental energy, awareness and introspection.

For this reason, dristis are also often used individually as tools in meditation practice. We therefore draw upon this meditative aspect to create tranquillity of mind and purity of inner vision, in order to reflect on our true nature as we move through the yogasanas.

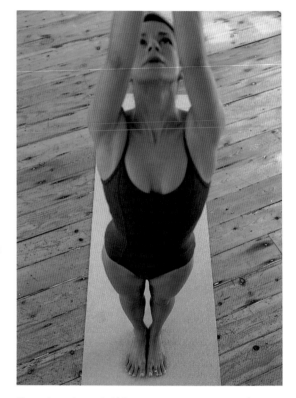

Above Angustha ma dyai (directing the focus to the thumbs) is the first dristi of Surya Namaskara (sun salutation).
Right Specific dristis being used to bring balance and focus.

Having a steady focal point also gives orientation and balance to the body in the postures, and helps to align the neck through the head position. The changes of dristi throughout Surya Namaskara (sun salutation) help the body's directional flow, cultivating physical and mental clarity. Dristis also strengthen the eye muscles and help to improve the eyesight – another practical physical benefit.

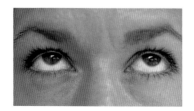

Above Dristi urdhva

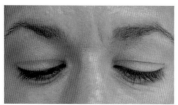

Above Dristi nasagrai

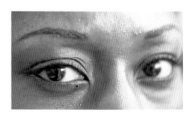

Above Dristi parsva

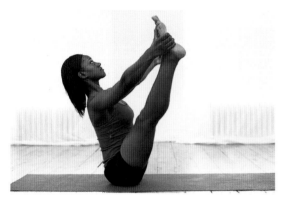

Above Dristi bhru madhya

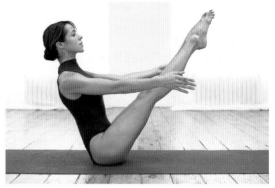

Above Dristi padhayoragrai

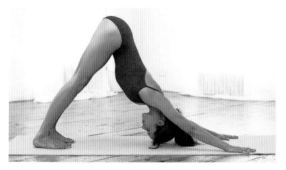

Above Dristi nabi chakra

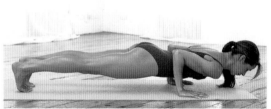

Above Dristi nasagrai

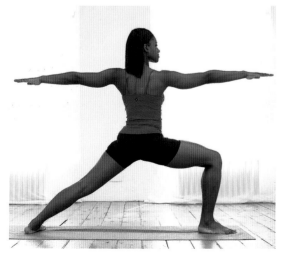

Above Dristi hastagrai

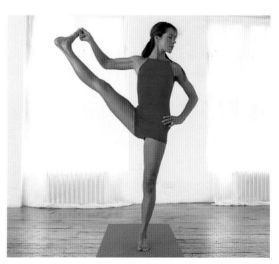

Above Dristi parsva

Preparing to Practise Astanga Yoga

Make yoga a part of your daily routine. Your practice is there to enhance your life rather than create stress, so don't worry if on some days you can't fit it in. However, regular, short practice sessions will be more beneficial than the occasional long session.

WHEN TO PRACTISE

- Traditionally, dawn and dusk are considered the most auspicious times of day to practise yoga, as the rising and setting of the sun both charge the atmosphere with spiritual energy. However, if these times are impossible for you, just practise when you can.

- Allow a minimum of three hours after a meal before you begin your practice. It is best to drink before and after your practice, so as not to become dehydrated, but avoid drinking during your practice, as this will interrupt your concentration and flow from one asana to another.

- Make time in your life for regular practice. Even if you can practise for only 15 minutes every other day, this is better than nothing at all. Over time, it is likely that you will want to give more time to your yoga, as your body and mind become revitalized by your practice.

HOW TO PRACTISE

- Never hold a posture – each asana is a moving, breathing experience, an exploration to open, release and strengthen your body and mind. The awakening journey of yoga is the goal, rather than the postures themselves.

- Always practise with awareness, care, attention and patience. Let your awareness extend not only to how you are breathing and moving but also to how you are thinking and feeling. Accept both good and bad thoughts and feelings equally with no judgement and no attachment, and then let them go as you breathe out, so that your yoga becomes a cleansing practice.

- Never push or bully your body to achieve a posture – injury will be sure to follow. Instead, allow yourself to flow with and yield to gravity. The natural force of gravity is far more powerful than ourselves, and if we surrender to it, it will take us deeper into the posture than any of our efforts using brute force.

- Always practise barefoot and wear soft, comfortable, non-restrictive clothing made of natural materials to allow your skin to breathe.

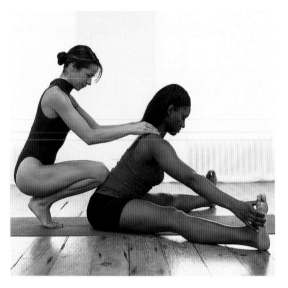

Above Gentle but firm hands-on adjustments can help the body to yield into asanas.

- Clear space for your practice – a clear, uncluttered space will help to create a clear, uncluttered mind.

- Practise systematically through the postures, starting with the sun salutes. With each session, add another posture and commit it to memory, so that you build your self-practice and carry it with you wherever you go.

- The three primary touchstones for you to be continuously aware of at all times are:

  1 The essence of your yoga practice – your breath. It will tell you when you are pushing too hard or when you have lost concentration. The breath is the link between body and mind, and a barometer to your state of being.
  2 Your foundations – your feet. Open and release them down into the ground to receive the upward surge of energy from the earth.
  3 The elongation of your spine – as you move through your practice, breathe length into your back to create space and energy within your body.

- Never confuse flow with rush. Flow steadily and smoothly through your postures, and this will generate dynamic energy, agility and awareness. Rushing through your practice will create a tense body and an agitated mind.

- Familiarize yourself with your body parts – in particular your feet, tailbone, sitting bones, pubic bone, sacrum, back ribs, collarbones, shoulder blades, neck, the crown of your head and the location of your three bandhas. Your bandhas need to be engaged throughout your practice, and throughout the instructions there are reminders.

- Always focus on breathing at lease five full, deep, steady breaths in each asana. As you develop strength, concentration and stamina, you may wish to take more breaths in order to sustain the postures for longer. Also, by breathing deeper and slower, you will create time and space to explore each asana fully.

- Before practising each posture, carefully study it by reading the instructions and observing the photographs to develop both a mental understanding and visual concept of it. Pay particular attention to the placement of the feet, as they are the foundation of each posture and the roots of your alignment.

- Shortened and moderated sequences are demonstrated in the chapter Abridged Sequences. As you become familiar and confident with the asanas and sequences you may wish to begin to develop your own practice, always closing with the key finishing asanas.

SAFETY IN PRACTICE
- Inversions (upside-down postures), jumps or any asana that feels strenuous should be avoided during recovery

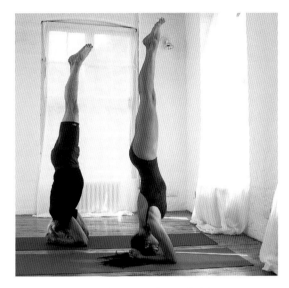

Above As you progress in your practice your body becomes stronger, more supple and agile.

from injury, during menstruation, or by those with high blood pressure, a hernia, a heart condition or a spinal injury such as prolapsed disc.

- Although many of the postures within this book are individually safe and extremely beneficial during pregnancy, the full Astanga primary series is unsuitable for expectant mothers and must not be practised in its complete form. Your yoga practice must be moderated during pregnancy; pre-natal yoga classes are recommended.

- The use of props such as straps, yoga blocks and cushions can be very useful when first learning an asana, or when recovering from injury, but it is unwise to become dependent on them. They are there initially to aid you rather than being a permanent crutch to your practice. A yoga mat, however, is one piece of equipment that you may wish to keep as your constant companion – they are light and easily transportable.

- Most importantly, enjoy your practice, and do not let it become a rigidly imposed ordeal. Instead, let yourself be creative, exploring the wonder of your body and its inner energy and wisdom. Listen to and respect your body, and let it lead you. It is your greatest teacher, and yoga is your inner sanctuary.

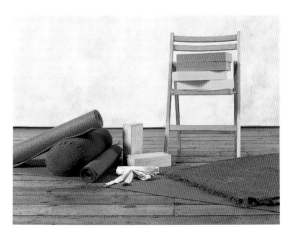

Above Chairs, foam blocks, wooden blocks, straps, bolsters and yoga mats are all props that can aid moderations of the asanas.

The Subtle Body

Within the subtle body there are energy channels called *nadis*. There are thought to be 72,000 such channels forming a complete network of energy pathways through which prana, the breath of life, flows, sustaining the physical body.

As breath also flows through the physical vessel of the manifest body, the breath is considered to be the vital link between the subtle and physical bodies. This is why the breath is the essence of our yoga practice, as it bridges the psychic and physical realms of our existence.

At the very core of the subtle body, and corresponding to the spine of the physical body, is the central spiritual channel of the sushumna nadi, *the most gracious channel*, along which there are seven energy centres, called chakras.

Weaving through the chakras and around the sushumna are two major subsidiary channels called *idi nadi*, the comforting channel, and *pingala nadi*, the tawny channel.

Pingala nadi stems from the right side of the sushumna nadi and is associated with the fiery, purifying energy of the sun, while ida nadi originates from the left of sushumna nadi and is associated with the soothing, cooling influence of the moon.

These two energy pathways feed into the sushumna through the chakras, where their dynamic polarities and opposing forces are integrated deep within the body.

On a physical level, these two nadis, like sushumna, have anatomical counterparts. Pingala nadi corresponds to the sympathetic (excitatory) nervous system, while ida nadi corresponds to the parasympathetic (relaxatory) nervous system.

On a spiritual level, our subtle body, the Sukshma-sharira, is believed to remain after death and is thought to be carried into future embodiment and reincarnation.

THE CHAKRAS

Chakra means "wheel or circle", and along the length of the sushumna nadi there are seven chakras. These chakras, which also correlate with key nerve centres or plexuses of the outer physical body, are like whirlpools of pranic energy, and each one signifies a different level of awareness. They are symbolic stepping-stones along the spiritual path.

Through the practice of the yoga postures, pranayama and meditation, the sushumna is cleansed, allowing pure energy to flow freely upwards through it, opening subtle dimensions of the mind and body to induce heightened states of consciousness and spiritual awakening.

This spiritual awakening is often depicted as a sleeping serpent coiled up at the base of the spine. As the snake is roused from its psychic slumber, serpent power (*kundalini-shakti*) is awakened, which activates the chakras as it

ascends through the sushumna, raising consciousness from the lower to the higher self.

CHAKRAS AND MEDITATION

The ancient art of meditation, the seventh limb of Astanga yoga, is known as dhyana and has been practised for thousands of years by many religions across the world. Dhyana is the process whereby the mind is freed from the restlessness of scattered thoughts in order to see clearly and look within to connect to our internal source of wisdom, happiness and divinity.

> The fabled musk deer searches the whole world over for the source of the scent which comes from within...
>
> Ramakrishna Paramhamsa

The mind is limitless, like the infinite blue expanse of the sky, but it is made small and foggy by our constant internal chatter of worries, anxieties, regrets, resentments, desires, memories, fantasies, dramas and set patterns of thinking. By releasing these clouds of thoughts, the unending open expansiveness of the inner mind and heart are revealed.

This opening into meditation is beyond words, and so, for this reason, meditation can only be experienced rather than taught. However, there are many wonderful techniques that help to induce meditative states. Be patient in your practice, as meditation will come in its own time when you are open to receive it.

Meditation is not an escape from the stresses and strains of everyday life. It is a meeting with the self in its fullness, and a living exploration of the wondrous life force within.

Primarily there are two categories of meditation: concrete, or *saguna* (with qualities), and abstract, or *nirguna* (without qualities). In saguna meditation, the mind contemplates and focuses on a concrete or definite object or image. In nirguna meditation, by contrast, there is no object; instead, the practitioner is absorbed in contemplating the absolute oneness of the universe. By focusing on the imagery of the chakras, heightened states of awareness can be induced. The image of the lotus is used to depict the chakras, because the lotus symbolizes the three stages of the spiritual journey:

1 The darkness of ignorance – the roots of the lotus grow in the dark, murky mud of swamps.
2 Aspiration – the stem of the lotus grows upwards away from the darkness towards the water's surface.
3 Illumination – as the lotus pierces the water's surface, its petals open up to the light of the sun, symbolizing spiritual enlightenment.

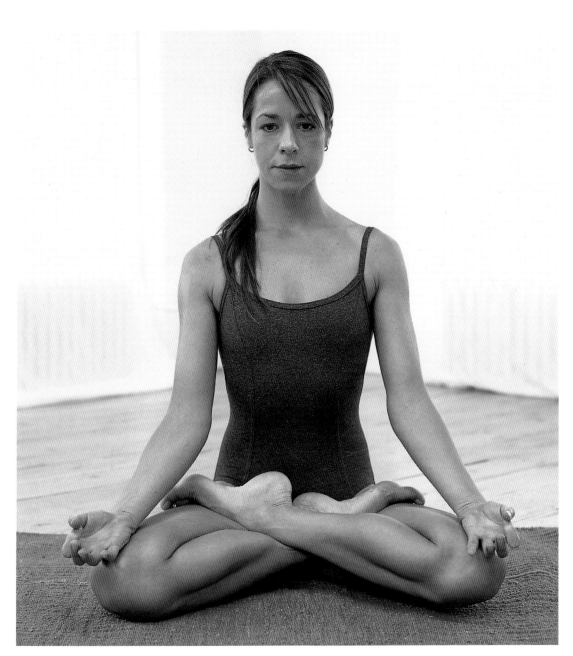

Above Sitting in Padmasana (lotus posture) encourages the body and mind to become still and steady. The folding of the legs creates a secure and firm foundation, providing the spine with a strong base to grow from. Steady stillness is the first step towards meditation. Curl your index finger under your thumb, symbolizing the individual self bowing to and uniting with the universal soul. This is called *chin mudra*.

Meditation

SITTING FOR MEDITATION

For the purpose of meditation, you must ensure that you assume a comfortable posture that you will be able to remain in without moving. Only when the body has been sitting in steady stillness for a while may meditation be experienced. Bring yourself to sit in any of the following asanas.

Sukhasana (easy happy posture)

Siddhasana (accomplished posture)

Ardha Padmasana (half lotus posture)

Padmasana (lotus posture as on the previous page)

Choose one in which you can comfortably maintain a straightness and length in your spine without feeling tension anywhere in your body. Sitting on a cushion or a yoga block is most useful in the beginning stages. As your back becomes stronger you will be able to sit for longer periods of time and without any props. If none of the above postures feels comfortable sit on a chair.

Once you have chosen your sitting position:

1 Sit evenly on both buttocks, so your foundation is balanced and steady.
2 Relax in your hips and legs, so your knees may release down towards the floor.
3 Lengthen your spine, drawing your back tall and long and your chest open.
4 Relax your shoulders, letting your arms release down and resting your hands on your knees.
5 Relax your face and jaw, gently lowering your chin slightly to bring length into the back of your neck.
6 Soften your eyes, lowering your focus or closing your eyes completely, and draw your awareness/consciousness to the natural flow and motion of your breath.

As you sit here in stillness, notice your chattering thoughts as they arise, but then simply observe them instead of getting caught up and trapped within the drama of them. Once you have noticed these thoughts clouding in, take a moment to breathe them all in. Don't get angry or frustrated by them, or try to suppress them, as this will cause you to get even further bound up with them all.

Let whatever needs to ripple up to the surface of your consciousness do so. See it, observe it, recognize it, feel it, and then slowly and gently breathe it all out, clearing your mind and returning your focus once more to the natural flow of your breathing.

As your mind becomes quieter and calmer, which may take some time and much practice at sitting, let your mind focus on the location, sensation, symbolic imagery and meaning of the various chakras.

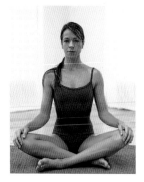
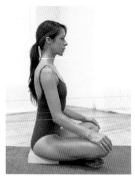

Above Sukhasana (easy happy posture) with and without a block.

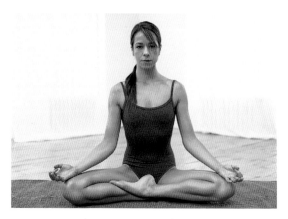

Above Siddhasana (accomplished posture)

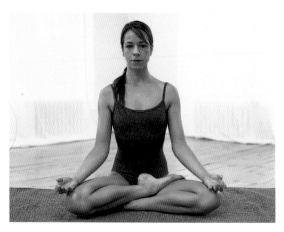

Above Ardha Padmasana (half lotus posture)

CHAKRAS: THEIR LOCATION, ELEMENT, IMAGERY AND MEANING

1 **Muladhara chakra** – root centre

mul = root or source; adhara = place or vital part

Muladhara chakra is the source of all energy available to humanity, whether it be physical, mental, emotional, spiritual or psychic. As this energy (known as kundalini-shakti) is released and drawn up through the chakras, it is purified, and spiritual awakening begins.

Physical location: perineum, pelvic plexus

Element: *prithvi tattva* (earth element)

Seed mantra: *lam*

Symbolism: a lotus flower of four deep-red petals. At the centre of the lotus flower is a glowing yellow square, representing the element of earth. Within the yellow square is an inverted red triangle, whose apex points downwards. This is shakti – the symbol of creative energy.

Internally focusing on the red triangle within the yellow square enhances inner balance and integration of creativity and stability.

2 **Svadhisthana chakra** – dwelling place of the self

sva = self or soul; adhisthana = abode or seat

This chakra is associated with relationships, procreation, pleasure and desire. It is the dwelling place of deep-rooted instincts and of all samskaras – mental and emotional impressions of the past.

Physical location: two finger widths above muladhara chakra and directly behind the genitals, hypogastric plexus

Element: *apas tattva* (water element)

Seed mantra: *vam*

Symbolism: a lotus flower of six deep-crimson petals. A bluey white crescent moon sits within the lower half of the lotus's circle, symbolizing the moon's influence on the ocean's tides and human emotion.

Concentrating on the image of a silvery blue crescent moon above a deep open ocean helps to restore emotional calm and balance desirous cravings. This helps in freeing us from compulsive behaviour and unhealthy habitual patterns of the past.

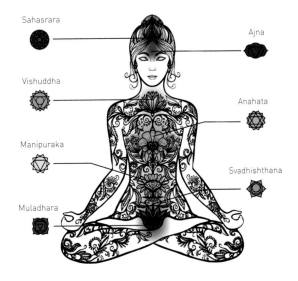

Above A depiction of the body's chakras and energy channels from an 18th-century manuscript.

Below Representations of the seven chakra centres and their symbolic imagery.

3 **Manipuraka chakra** – city of jewels

mani = gem or jewel; puraka = city

Manipuraka chakra is the centre of inner power, energy, ambitious drive and assertiveness.

Physical location: situated behind the navel, solar plexus

Element: *agni tattva* (fire element)

Seed mantra: *ram*

Symbolism: a lotus flower of ten petals. Within the circle of the lotus is a downward-pointing fiery red triangle, like a gleaming ruby signifying energy and power.

Visualizing golden light radiating out from the fiery triangle and spreading throughout the body cultivates physical, mental and psychic energy, dynamism and vitality.

| 1 Muladhara chakra | 2 Svadhishthana chakra | 3 Manipuraka chakra | 4 Anahata chakra | 5 Vishuddha chakra | 6 Ajna chakra | 7 Sahasrara chakra |

4 **Anahata chakra** – unstruck sound

anahata = unstruck, referring to cosmic sound, which does not arise from two objects being struck (as with all other sounds) but is always present in the heart

From this centre the internal vibration and pulsing of the heart can be heard, sending out waves of compassion, unconditional love and understanding of equality and brotherhood.

Physical location: behind the sternum, level with the heart (for this reason this chakra is often called the "lotus of the heart"), cardiac plexus

Element: *vaya tattva* (air element)

Seed mantra: *yam*

Symbolism: a lotus flower of 12 petals. At the centre of the lotus is a star of six points like a hexagram, which is created by two triangles interlacing, one with an apex pointing up and the other with one pointing down. The upward and downward triangles denote the midway balance of the lower chakras of physical existence and the upper chakras of spiritual and transcendental levels. Within the star there is a gentle burning flame – the symbol of the individual soul (jiva).

Focusing on the steadiness of the inner flame of the heart connects us to our individual soul, internal truth and compassion, which remain steady and undisturbed by the external activities of the world.

5 **Vishuddha chakra** – wheel of purity

shuddi = purification

It is at this centre that all dualities, polarities and dichotomies of opposites are accepted within ourselves without judgement.

Physical location: behind the well of the throat, pharyngeal plexus

Element: *akasha tattva* (ether element)

Seed mantra: *ham*

Symbolism: a lotus flower of 16 violet petals. Within the lotus flower is a white circle like a silvery full moon, with a teardrop shape of nectar at its centre, symbolizing the harmonizing and purifying of all polarities and opposites.

Visualizing and sensing a sweet teardrop of nectar, like calming balm at the level of the throat as you breathe, is said to help smooth internal conflicts of heart and mind. This helps to cultivate understanding and a non-judgemental attitude to mind and heart.

6 **Ajna chakra** – command centre

ajni = command

This energy centre is the gateway to our intuition, where communication and command from the internal guru is heard. At this point the link between the mental and psychic aspects of our being is created as the three channels of sushumna, ida and pingala converge.

Physical location: behind the space in between the eyebrows, mid-brain at the medulla and pineal plexuses. Because of its location at the third eye it may also be referred to as *jnana chakshu* – the eye of wisdom.

Element: *maha tattva* (cause of the mind element)

Seed mantra: *om*

Symbolism: a two-petalled silver lotus, one petal representing the sun (pingala) and one the moon (ida). The circle of the lotus is of a silvery white shade, with a lingam (symbol of masculine creative energy) in its centre, placed within a downward-pointing triangle, which is a symbol of the feminine principle (shakti).

Focusing on a glowing circle of light at the centre of your eyebrows, radiating wisdom and intuition, enhances insight and inner knowing.

7 **Sahasrara chakra** – thousand petalled lotus

sahasrara = thousand-spoked; also known as sunya, the voidless void of totality

This is not really a chakra, but the dwelling place of our highest awareness. It is the union of all consciousness and all energy.

Physical location: crown of the head, top of the skull

Seed mantra: entire Sanskrit alphabet

Symbolism: a circular lotus blossom of a thousand shining petals overlying one another. Inscribed on each petal is a letter (*matrika*) of the Sanskrit alphabet. In the centre of the lotus is a full moon (*purna chandra*), and within the full moon is a *jyotirlinga* – a lingam of light shining upwards, symbolizing pure consciousness.

It is said that the experience of sahasrara is beyond words and all definition – it has to be felt to be understood. Practitioners of different religions describe it in different words: Christians refer to it as heaven, the Buddhists call it nirvana, yogis name it as samadhi and Hindus call it *kaivalya*. It is the perfect merging of all things – it is yoga itself.

Right The seven chakras along the central energy channel of the sushumna with the intertwining ida nadi (moon energy) stemming from the left side, and the pingala nadi (sun energy) from the right.

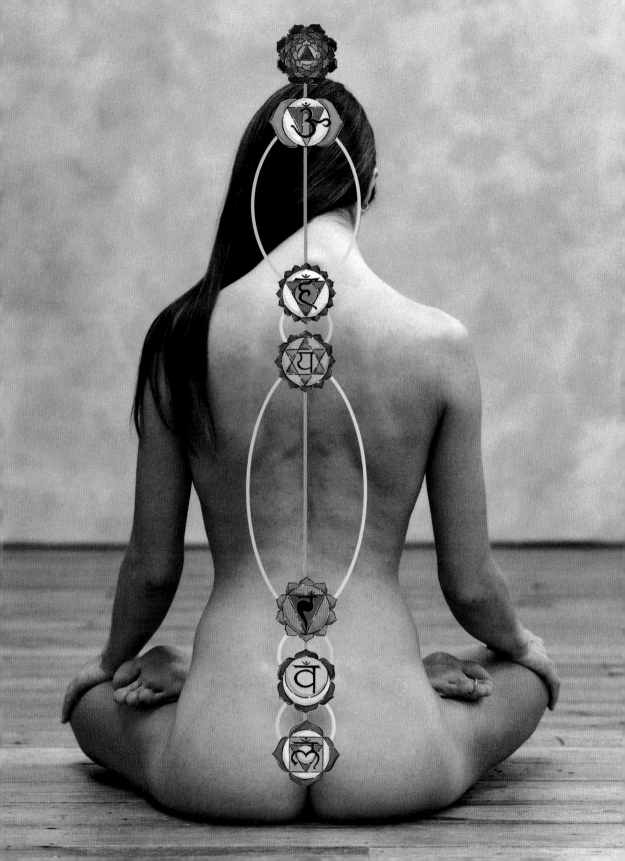

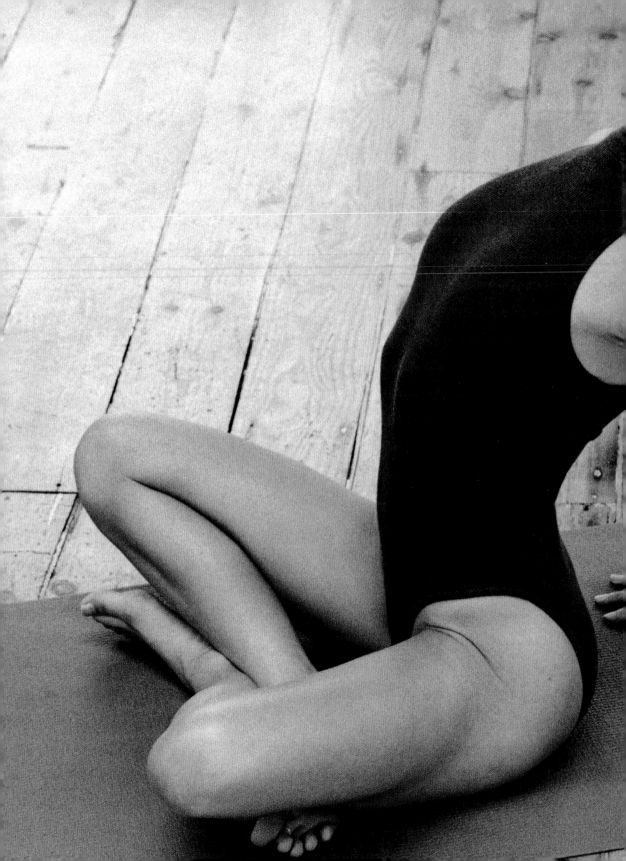

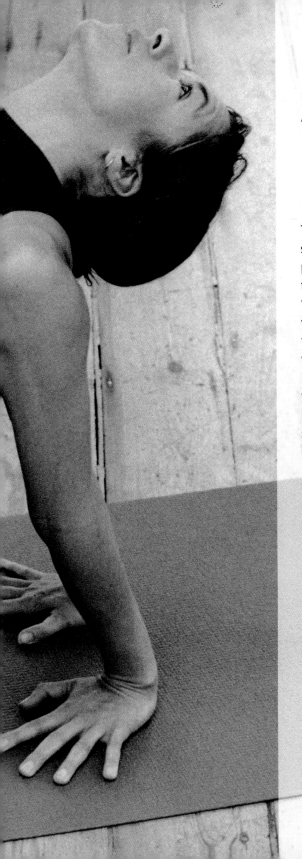

The Primary Series

The Yoga Korunta consists of six series of some forty postures each. The first series, or primary series, is called Yoga Chikitsa (yoga therapy). It is sometimes referred to as the "healing series", as the asanas (postures) within it realign, rebalance and cleanse both the body and the mind, restoring health and vitality. The second series or intermediate level, is called Nadi Sodhana (purification of the subtle channels). It works on harmonizing body and mind by fortifying the nervous system. The advanced series, 3rd, 4th, 5th and 6th, develop and intensify vital prana energy.

This book focuses on the first series. Through Surya Namaskara A and B (sun salutations), the body–breath–mind connection is awakened. The standing asanas develop concentration and strength; the seated asanas create suppleness and a sense of calm; and the finishing sequence slows the mind, cultivating clarity and a meditative state.

Yoga Chikitsa

In this chapter the flow form of the primary series is shown in its entirety, leading you through the correct sequential order of asanas. By steadily progressing through the postures you will gain strength, flexibility and a deepened understanding of your body and mind, which will help guide you along the yogic path.

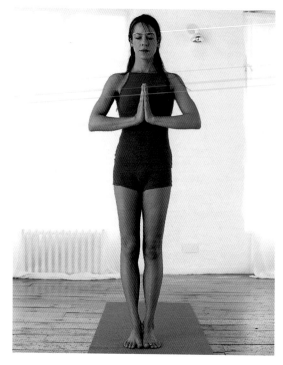

Above While standing in Tadasana, bring the palms together in namaste and recite your mantra at the beginning of a practice.

Once the primary series is mastered, progression on to the second series, Nadi Sodhana, and eventually the advanced series, follows. It is a natural journey that will unfold with time and practice. There is no need to hurry, as the asanas and the series are purely a vehicle by which you may access your soul.

THE MANTRA

The yoga mantra is spoken at the beginning and end of practice, usually in the original Sanskrit. It should be repeated with an openness of mind to absorb its full meaning which will become more apparent with time.

Mantras are subtle resonation structures and sacred phrases expressing intention and thought as sound, in much the same way as a prayer. They are the link between consciousness and manifest sound, and have far-reaching powers of transformation, turning negative impulses into positive ones and heightening realms of awareness through their sound vibration.

It is auspicious to open and close your yoga practice with a mantra, and the one at the foot of this page is traditional. Alternatively reciting silently or aloud the syllable of OM ॐ (the primordial sound, seed of creation and all mantras) will help to channel the body's energy and focus the mind. OM forms part of all mantras, is spelt AUM in Sanskrit. Each letter is a sacred symbol:

A represents the individual physical self in the material world
U represents the psychic realms of the mind
M represents the in-dwelling spiritual light of the intuitive self

Repeating this OM mantra for 20 minutes relaxes every atom of the body.

OPENING ASTANGA YOGA MANTRA

~OM~
VANDE GURŪṆĀM CARAṆĀRAVINDE
SANDARIŚITA SVĀTMA SUKHĀVA BODHE
NIḤ ŚREYASE JĀṄGALIKĀYAMĀNE
SAMSĀRA HĀLĀ HALA MOHAŚĀNTYAI

ĀBĀHU PURUṢĀKĀRAM
ŚAṄKHACAKRĀSI DHĀRIAM
SAHASRA ŚIRASAM ŚVETAM
PRAṆAMĀMI PATAÑJALIM
~OM~

TRANSLATION

I pray to the lotus feet of the supreme guru
Awakening the happiness of the inner self revealed
Acting like a doctor of the jungle
Able to pacify the delusion of the poison of conditioned existence

To Patanjali, incarnate of Adisesa, white in colour with 1000
    glowing heads of the divine serpent Anata,
Human in form carrying the sword of discrimination,
    the eternal wheel of fire and light and a conch of divine sound,
I prostrate

SURYA NAMASKARA A

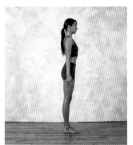

Tadasana Mountain posture p44

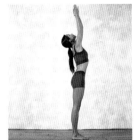

Urdhva Tadasana Upward mountain posture p44

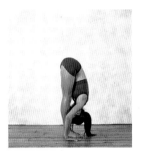

Uttanasana Intense stretch posture p44

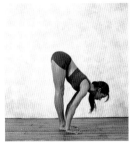

Urdhva Uttanasana Upwards intense stretch posture p44

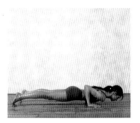

Chaturanga Dandasana Four limbs staff posture p45

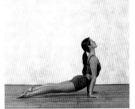

Urdhva Mukha Svanasana Upward facing dog p45

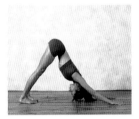

Adho Mukha Svanasana Downward facing dog p45

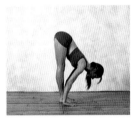

Urdhva Uttanasana Upward intense stretch posture p45

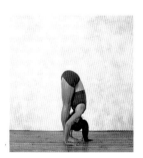

Uttanasana Intense stretch posture p46

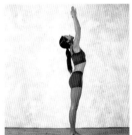

Urdhva Tadasana Upward mountain posture p46

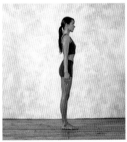

Tadasana Mountain posture p46

SURYA NAMASKARA B

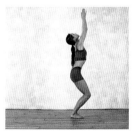

Utkatasana Powerful posture p47

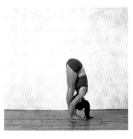

Uttanasana Intense stretch posture p47

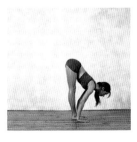

Urdhva Uttanasana Upwards intense stretch posture p47

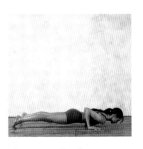

Chaturanga Dandasana Four limbs staff posture p47

▷

SURYA NAMASKARA B CONTINUED

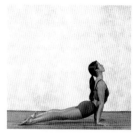

Urdhva Mukha Svanasana
Upward facing dog p47

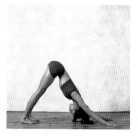

Adho Mukha Svanasana
Downward facing dog p47

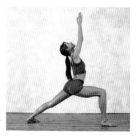

Virabhadrasana I Warrior
posture I p48

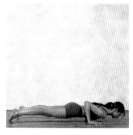

Chaturanga Dandasana
Four limbs staff posture p48

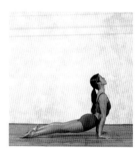

Urdhva Mukha Svanasana
Upward facing dog p48

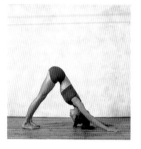

Adho Mukha Svanasana
Downward facing dog p48

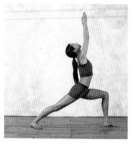

Virabhadrasana I Warrior
posture I p48

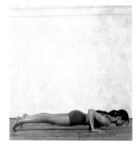

Chaturanga Dandasana
Four limbs staff posture p48

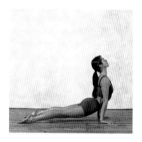

Urdhva Mukha Svanasana
Upward facing dog p49

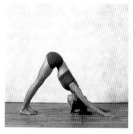

Adho Mukha Svanasana
Downward facing dog p49

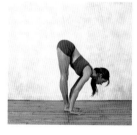

Urdhva Uttanasana Upward
intense stretch posture p49

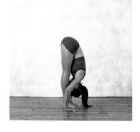

Uttanasana Intense stretch
posture p49

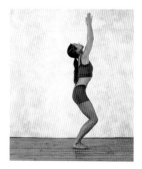

Utkatasana Powerful
posture p49

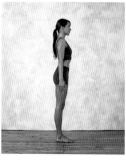

Tadasana Mountain
posture p49

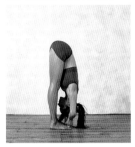

Padangusthasana Foot big toe posture p50

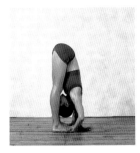

Pada Hastasana Foot hand posture p51

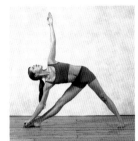

Utthita Trikonasana Extended triangle p52

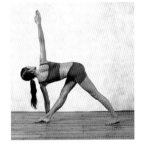

Parivrtta Trikonasana Revolved triangle p53

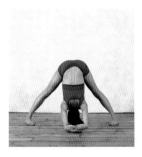

Utthita Parsvakonasana Extended lateral angle p54

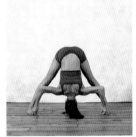

Parivrtta Parsvakonasana Revolved lateral angle p55

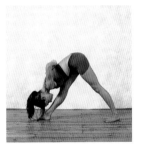

Prasarita Padottanasana A Expanded leg stretch A p56

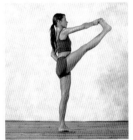

Prasarita Padottanasana B Expanded leg stretch B p57

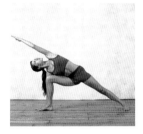

Prasarita Padottanasana C Expanded leg stretch C p58

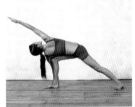

Prasarita Padottanasana D Expanded leg stretch D p59

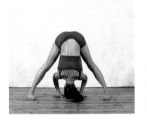

Parsvottanasana Side Intense stretch posture p60

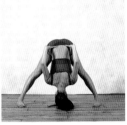

Utthita Hasta Padangusthasana Extended hand big toe p61

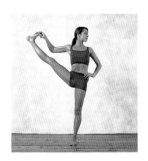

Utthita Parsvasahita A Extended side posture p62

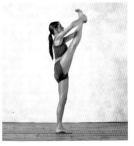

Utthita Parsvasahita B Extended side posture p63

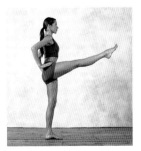

Utthita Parsvasahita C Extended side posture p63

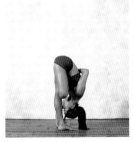

Ardha Baddha Padmottanasana half bound lotus stretch p64

▷

STANDING POSTURES CONTINUED

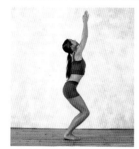

Utkatasana Powerful posture p65

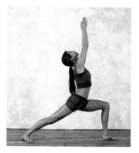

Virabhadrasana I Warrior posture I p66

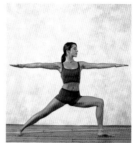

Virabhadrasana II Warrior posture II p67

SEATED POSTURES

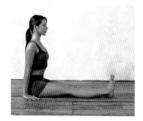

Dandasana Staff posture p72

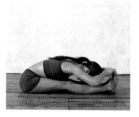

Paschimottanasana A Stretch of the West A p72

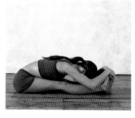

Paschimottanasana B Stretch of the West B p73

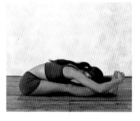

Paschimottanasana C Stretch of the West C p73

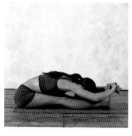

Paschimottanasana D Stretch of the West D p73

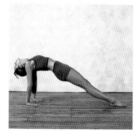

Purvottansana Stretch of the East p76

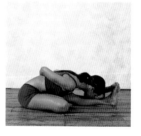

Ardha Baddha Padma Paschimottanasana Half bound lotus stretch p77

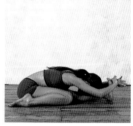

Triang Mukhaikapada Paschimottanasana Three limbs face one leg stretch p78

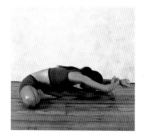

Janu Sirsasana A Knee head posture A p79

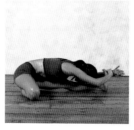

Janu Sirsasana B Knee head posture B p80

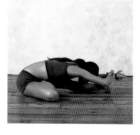

Janu Sirsasana C Knee head posture C p81

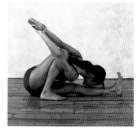

Marichyasana A Sage Marichi posture A p82

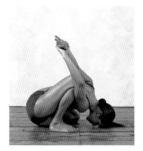

Marichyasana B Sage
Marichi posture B p83

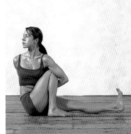

Marichyasana C Sage
Marichi posture C p84

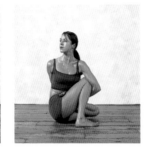

Marichyasana D Sage
Marichi posture D p85

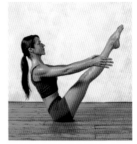

Navasana Boat posture p86

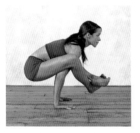

Bhujapidasana A Arm
pressure posture A p87

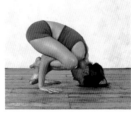

Bhujapidasana B Arm
pressure posture B p87

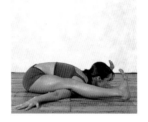

Kurmasana Tortoise
posture p89

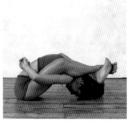

Supta Kurmasana Sleeping
tortoise posture p90

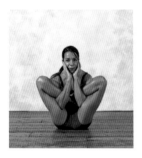

Garbha Pindasana Womb
embryo posture p92

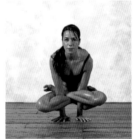

Kukkutasana Rooster
posture p93

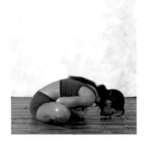

Baddha Konasana A Bound
angle posture A p94

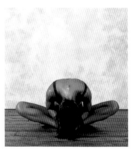

Baddha Konasana B Bound
angle posture B p94

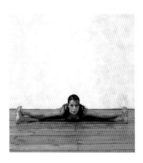

Upavista Konasana A Seated
angle posture A p95

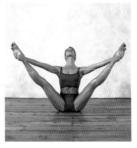

Upavista Konasana B Seated
angle posture B p96

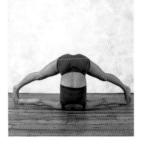

Supta Konasana A Sleeping
angle posture A p97

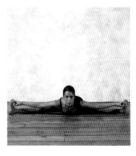

Supta Konasana B Sleeping
angle posture B p98

▷

SEATED POSTURES CONTINUED

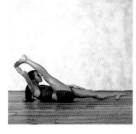

Supta Padangusthasana
Sleeping foot big toe p99

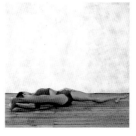

Supta Parsvasahita A
Sleeping side posture A p100

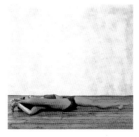

Supta Parsvasahita B
Sleeping side posture B p101

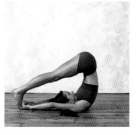

Ubhaya Padangusthasana A
Both feet big toe posture A p103

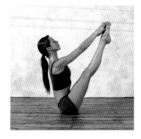

Ubhaya Padangusthasana B
Both feet big toe posture B
p103

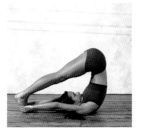

**Urdhva Mukha
Paschimottanasana A**
Upward facing stretch A p104

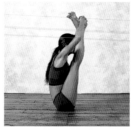

**Urdhva Mukha
Paschimottanasana B**
Upward facing stretch B p104

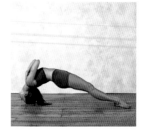

Setu Bandhasana Bridge
posture p105

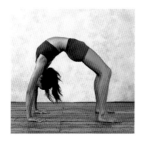

Urdhva Dhanurasana
Upward bow posture p106

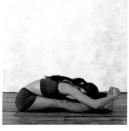

Paschimottanasana C
Stretch of the West C p73

FINISHING SEQUENCE

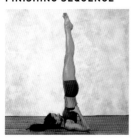

Salamba Sarvangasana
Supported body posture p112

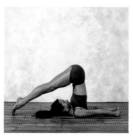

Halasana Plough
posture p114

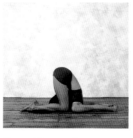

Karnapidasana Ear pressure
posture p115

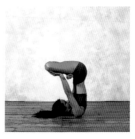

Urdhva Padmasana Upward
lotus posture p116

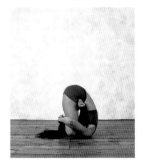

Pindasana Embryo posture p117

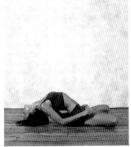

Matsyasana Fish posture p118

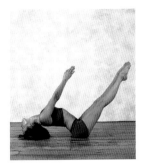

Uttana Padasana Extended feet posture p119

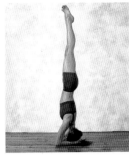

Sirsasana Headstand posture p120

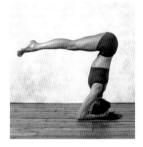

Sirsasana Urdhva Dandasana Headstand upward staff p123

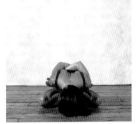

Yoga Mudrasana Yoga sealing posture p125

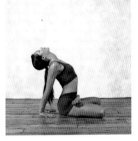

Padmasana A Lotus posture A p126

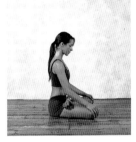

Padmasana B Lotus posture B p126

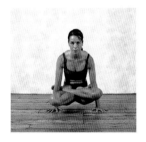

Tolasana Scales posture p127

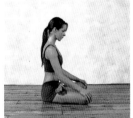

Padmasana Lotus posture p126

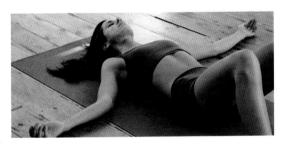

Savasana/Mrtasana Corpse posture p128

CLOSING ASTANGA YOGA MANTRA

~OM~
SWASTHI – PRAJĀ BHYAH PARI PALA YANTAM
NYĀ – YENA MĀRGENA MAHI – MAHISHĀHA
GO – BRĀHMANEBHYAHA – SHUBHAMASTU –
  NITYAM
LOKĀA – SAMASTHĀ SUKHINO – BHAVANTHU
~OM~

TRANSLATION

Let prosperity be glorified
May law and justice rule the world
May all divinity be protected and
May people of the whole world be happy and prosperous

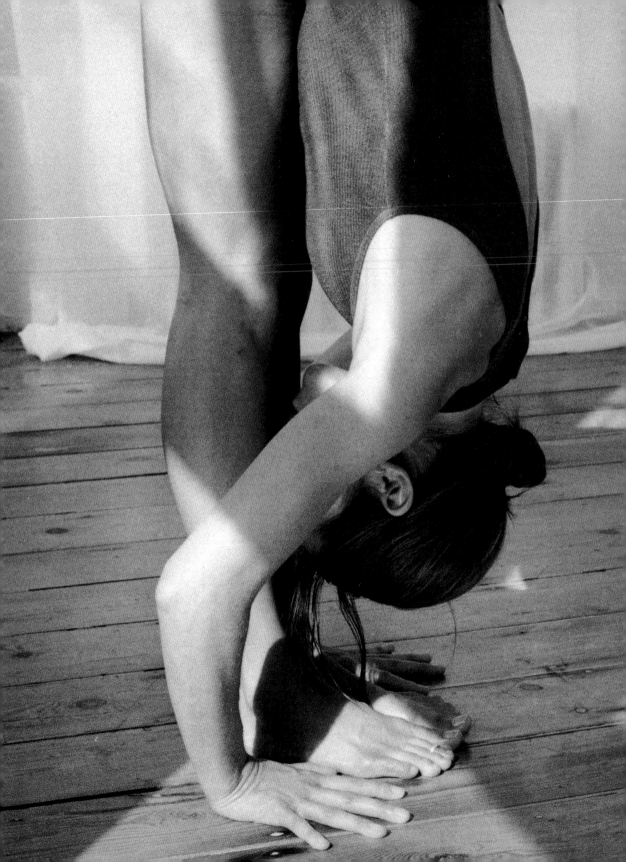

Standing Asanas

Yoga Chikitsa, the primary series, begins
by standing in the stillness of Tadasana.
As you move through Surya Namaskara
and the following asanas, the feet open into
the ground, discovering a sound relationship
with the earth. At the same time, the vital
energy of your breath surges up from the
ground, imbuing your entire body and yoga
postures with life.

Surya Namaskara serves to warm and
awaken the body before moving forwards in
the standing postures. The standing asanas
align the body to develop strength, stamina
and tone.

At the end of the standing sequence we
return to the inspiration of Surya Namaskara
to create a vinyasa flow through the last
standing postures. From here a linking jump
leads us directly into the seated asanas.

Tāḍāsana/Samasthiti | MOUNTAIN POSTURE

tada = mountain
sama = upright
sthiti = still and steady

Through the practice of Tadasana the body is released from bad posture and develops clear alignment through the skeleton. This creates vitality, health and balance within the body, providing the opportunity for standing strong without carrying tension.

1 Stand quietly at the front of your yoga mat with your feet together, feeling the skin of your big-toe joints, inner heels and ankle bones touching. Soften the soles of your feet into the floor and let your toes open out like roots.

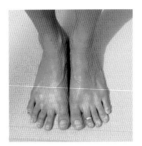

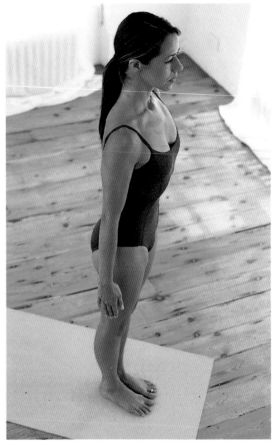

2 Draw your focus inwards, internalizing your awareness, and begin to relax within this standing stillness. Do not tense your muscles, just *breathe softly* and fully, feeling gravity flowing down from the back of your waist through into your tailbone and legs, allowing your weight to drop evenly through your feet into the floor. At the same time, feel energy gently streaming up through your spine, lengthening along the back of your neck and allowing the crown of your skull to float skywards.

With an internal focus, align your hips over your feet and ankles, allowing your sitting bones to release down over your heel bones. Open your shoulders, feeling them directly placed over your pelvis, and balance your head on top of your neck, keeping your throat soft. Allow your bones to fall into alignment without muscular force or tension, which would block the flow of energy and prevent the natural alignment of your skeleton.

In this way, you align from within, stacking your major joints (ankles, knees, hips and shoulders) one above the other like building blocks. Your kneecaps must always follow the same direction as your toes.

The first building block of yoga

All the standing yoga asanas are born out of Tadasana, and it is from this point of standing in the stillness of mountain posture that the sun salutations begin. Tadasana teaches us how to be still and at ease as we stand alone on our own two feet, and so is central to our practice. As you begin to learn Tadasana, it is important to focus on your internal skeleton, as your bones are the roots of alignment and correct posture. In order for this deep alignment to take place, you need to relax your skin, muscles, mind and heart. By aligning your bones, structural stability and harmony are created from within. Core strength is developed and the muscles can then follow and draw up to support that stability, harmony and movement of your body.

As you stand in Tadasana, allow your mind to become quiet. The quieter we become, the more able we are to listen to, and deepen our awareness of the energies flowing through our body and existence.

The breath brings new life to these energies, and with the quietness of mind and stillness of body a connection to the rhythmic flow of our breath is made. This connection is our constant backdrop and the inspiration for all existence, which carries and moves us from the inside out through our life and yoga practice.

With improved posture comes ease of movement, confidence, the release of compression on bones and joints, and the creation of internal space for our organs to sit correctly and our lungs to breathe fully.

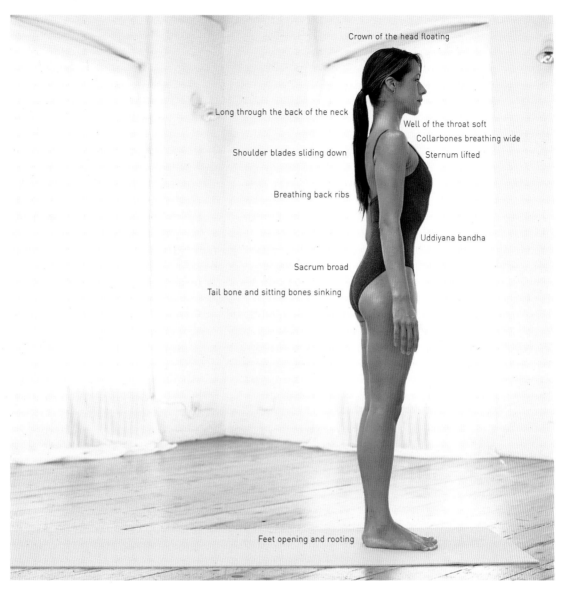

Crown of the head floating

Long through the back of the neck

Well of the throat soft
Collarbones breathing wide
Sternum lifted

Shoulder blades sliding down

Breathing back ribs

Uddiyana bandha

Sacrum broad

Tail bone and sitting bones sinking

Feet opening and rooting

3 Now take your awareness to your perineum and engage mula bandha without gripping your buttocks. Draw your lower abdomen upwards and in, connecting to uddiyana bandha, and softly release your shoulders down and wide. Gently draw in your throat muscles, engaging jalandhara bandha, and guide your breath into ujjayi breathing.

Let your muscles draw in on to your bones, supporting your internal alignment. As you *breathe*, grow into stillness, feeling the subtle internal motion of your breath – both the rising energy of your inhalation (prana) opening you into space, and the down-flowing energy of your exhalation (*aparna*) centring you into the ground.

Once you are in Tadasana
Be aware of and continue the following:
• body breathing
• releasing and opening the feet into the ground
• feeling rebounding energy flowing up through your spine
• yielding the shoulders, tailbone and heels to gravity
• breathing in the sky and breathing it back out again

From breathing in Tadasana, the sequences of Surya Namaskara begin, with each breath moving your body into and out of each asana.

Surya Namaskara A | SUN SALUTATION A

surya = sun
namaskara = respectful greeting
or salute

The flowing sequence of asanas within Surya Namaskara warms and primes the body, building upon the alignment created in Tadasana. With each repetition, prana is generated, helping to deepen awareness and expand consciousness into the practice.

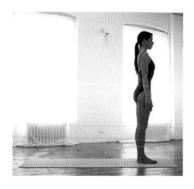

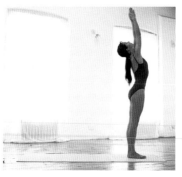

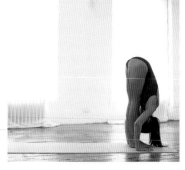

1 TADASANA (mountain posture) Start by quietly standing in this pose. Feel the steady stillness of Tadasana and start to listen to your *breath*, becoming aware of its natural rhythm, and then allow ujjayi pranayama to begin to flow.

2 URDHVA TADASANA (upward mountain posture) *Take a deep inhalation*, as you open your arms out to the sides, stretching up, bringing your palms together into a high prayer gesture. Let energy rise up through your waist to your fingertips and at the same time slide your shoulders and tailbone down wards opening the soles of your feet into the floor. Lift your gaze up to your thumbs, <u>dristi</u>: angustha ma dyai.

3 UTTANASANA (intense stretch posture) *Slowly exhale*, and fold deeply over your legs. Place your hands on the floor on either side of your feet, and let your head drop down, <u>dristi</u>: nasagrai.

Moderation If your fingers cannot reach the floor with your legs straight, place your hands on your ankles.

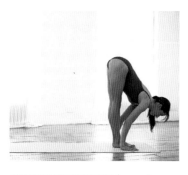

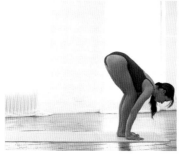

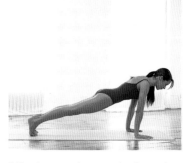

4 URDHVA UTTANASANA (upwards intense stretch posture). *Inhale* lifting and opening your chest and heart forwards as you root your feet downwards. Lengthen through your back, keeping your neck long and in line with your spine. Draw the crown of your head forwards and your shoulder blades down your back. Keep your hands on the floor or ankles. Focus along the nose tip, <u>dristi</u>: nasagrai.

5 PREPARING TO JUMP BACK *Retain your breath*, and bend your knees, keeping your chest lifted and your spine stretching long. Place your hands at the sides of your feet on the floor, if they are not there already, and spread your palms open, pressing them down into the ground. Extend your fingers, with your middle fingers stretching forwards.

6 Keeping your chest opening forwards, softly jump your feet back, allowing them to part slightly. Make sure your shoulders remain aligned over your hands. Feel the body straight and strong in this plank-like position, but do not stay here. Instead, move on smoothly to step 7. Step back if you do not feel confident to jump.

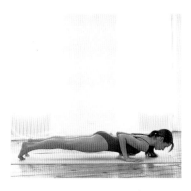

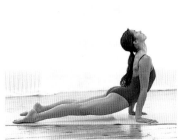

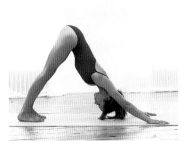

7 CHATURANGA DANDASANA (four limbs staff posture) *Exhale*, bend your elbows, drawing them close into the sides of your body, and lower yourself towards the floor. Keep your spine long and your body straight and parallel to the floor. Broaden your shoulders, engage uddiyana bandha and hover 5cm/2in off the floor. Keep your toes active, pressing into the floor as they are tucked under, spread your palms open and down. Look towards your nose, <u>dristi</u>: **nasagrai**.

8 URDHVA MUKHA SVANASANA (upward facing dog posture) *Inhale*, pushing with your toes so that they are stretch long, lift your chest and face skywards, arching up evenly through your spine. Gently roll your inner arms forwards and in towards the sides of your waist, without locking the elbows. Draw your shoulders back and stretch your legs long. Press the front of your feet and your palms down into the floor, so that the shins, knees, and thighs do not touch the floor, <u>dristi</u>: **nasagrai**.

9 ADHO MUKHA SVANASANA (downward facing dog posture) *Exhale*, roll over the front of your toes and push your hips and buttock bones up and back. Align your feet hip-width apart and extend the outer edges of your feet down while pressing open your big-toe joints into the floor. Spread your toes and fingers, and plant your palms into your mat. Release your shoulders wide, sliding the blades up your back, and gently press your chest towards your legs. Draw your thigh muscles up and on to your upper thigh bones. Sink your heels down into the floor to send your sitting bones higher up. Move your chin in to bring length into the back of your neck, <u>dristi</u>: **nabi chakra**. *Take five long, deep breaths*, gathering energy.

Moderation Try bending your knees and lowering your chest in between your hands, keeping the hips lifted.

Moderation Allow your knees to rest on the floor until you gradually build up the strength to work the full pose.

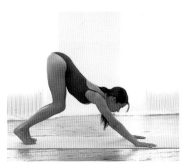

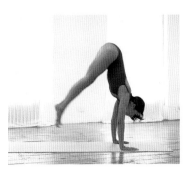

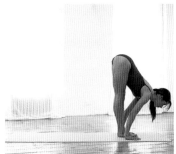

10 JUMP INTO URDHVA UTTANASANA Towards the end of your fifth exhalation, shift your head and shoulders forwards over your hands, allowing your knees to bend slightly and your heels to lift a little off the floor. Keeping your hips well lifted, and still drawing your focus forwards, rock back on to the balls of your feet, bending your knees still further.

11 As you *inhale*, rebound off your toes and lightly jump, projecting your hips upwards and your feet forwards and together in between your hands. At first you may want to step your feet in, especially if you have knee or back injuries.

12 As your feet touch down, keep a lift in your chest and stretch through your spine.

Moderation Place your hands on your ankles and bend your knees, as you stretch your spine forwards.

▷

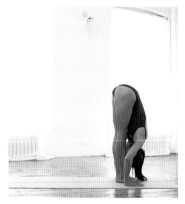

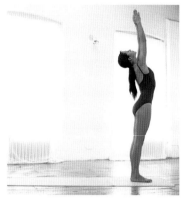

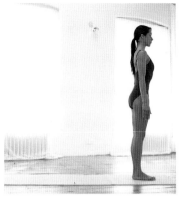

13 UTTANASANA (intense stretch posture) *Slowly and completely exhale*, folding deeply over from your hips. Bring your torso in towards your thighs, and extend the crown of your head down. Make sure your feet are together and that your neck and shoulders are relaxed. Look along your nose tip, <u>dristi</u>: **nasagrai**, and move your chin in towards your chest.

Moderation If you feel any back strain, protect your back by bending your knees and placing your hands on your ankles.

14 URDHVA TADASANA (upward mountain posture) *Inhale*, lifting up through your abdomen and back while pressing your feet firmly into the ground. Raise your arms sideways, bringing your palms together overhead into Urdhva Tadasana. Lift your chest and gaze up to your thumbs and skywards, <u>dristi</u>: **angustha ma dyai**.

15 TADASANA (mountain posture) *Exhale* and turn the palms downwards as you lower your arms down by the sides of your body. Feel your spine lengthening up into Tadasana, and open the soles of your feet broad into the floor beneath you.

• Repeat five to eight times, then move on to Surya Namaskara B

The importance of Surya Namaskara
• The sun salutation connects body, mind and breath, setting the correct tone and atmosphere to begin your yoga practice. It signifies the worship of the sun god – provider of health and vitality – and is traditionally performed as the sun rises at the dawn of a new day.

• Joints are softly opened, muscles gently stretched, internal organs massaged and the mind–body–breath connection awakened, preparing you for the following journey through the primary series of asanas.

• As the breath and body flow together, an internal heat is created. This begins a process of purification, burning toxins as they are drawn out from the organs, joints and muscles and released through the skin as perspiration.

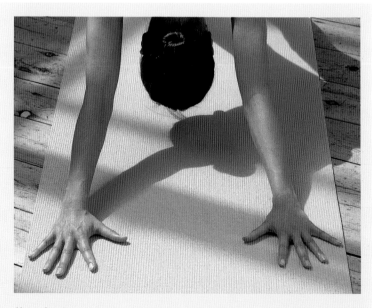

Above Opening your hands generously into the floor with your middle finger stretching forwards develops a secure base in downward facing dog posture.

Sūrya Namaskara B | SUN SALUTATION B

surya = sun
namaskara = respectful greeting
or salute

This second sun salute builds on the first, introducing the posture of Virabhadrasana I (warrior I). This intensifies the internal heat of the body, develops physical stamina and creates a powerful co-ordination of the breath and body in motion.

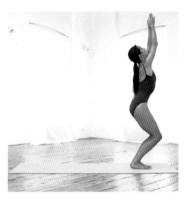

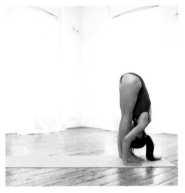

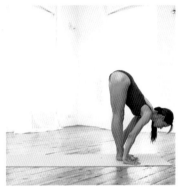

1 UTKATASANA (powerful posture) From Surya Namaskara A, *inhale*, bend your knees deeply and soften at the front of your ankles. Raise your arms sideways and join your palms together arrowing your fingers upwards. Sit your hips low and draw your shoulder blades down your back, raising your focus up to your thumbs, <u>dristi</u>: **angustha ma dyai**.

2 UTTANASANA (intense stretch posture), as in Surya Namaskara A. *Exhale.*

3 URDHVA UTTANASANA (upward intense stretch posture), as in Surya Namaskara A. *Inhale.* Followed by bending your knees to prepare to jump back.

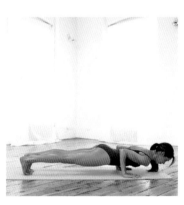

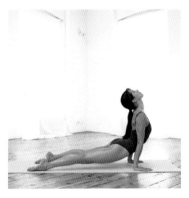

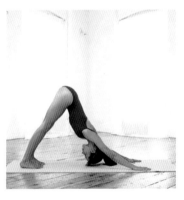

4 CHATURANGA DANDASANA (four limbs staff posture), as in Surya Namaskara A. *Exhale.*

5 URDHVA MUKHA SVANASANA (upward facing dog posture), as in Surya Namaskara A. *Inhale.*

6 ADHO MUKHA SVANASANA (downward facing dog posture), as in Surya Namaskara A. *Exhale.*

Moderation Allow your knees to bend but still focus on tilting your pelvis forwards and your buttocks up.

▷

STANDING ASANAS

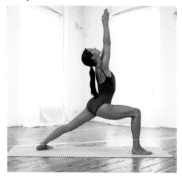

7 VIRABHADRASANA I (warrior posture I) Pivoting on the ball of your left foot, rotate your left heel in and forwards by 45 degrees towards the arch of your right foot. *Inhale slowly* and step your right foot forwards in between your hands, placing it in line with your right hip. Bend your right knee deeply, drawing it over your ankle, while pressing the sole of your left foot firmly into the floor. Lift up your body, lengthen through your spine and open your arms sideways and then overhead, bringing the palms together. Relax your shoulders and open your chest and face upwards, <u>dristi</u>: **angustha ma dyai.**

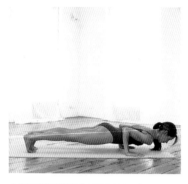

8 CHATURANGA DANDASANA (four limbs staff posture) *Exhale*, placing your hands on the ground on either side of your right foot. Keeping your hips low and your shoulders aligned directly over your hands, take your right foot back parallel to the left and lower yourself down into Chaturanga Dandasana. Look down along the nose tip towards the floor, <u>dristi</u>: **nasagrai.**

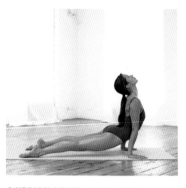

9 URDHVA MUKHA SVANASANA (upward facing dog posture) as in Surya Namaskara A. *Inhale.*

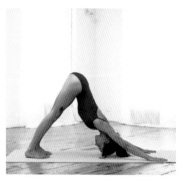

10 ADHO MUKHA SVANASANA (downward facing dog posture) *Exhale*, roll over your toes and lift your hips up and back into Adho Mukha Svanasana. Look towards your navel, <u>dristi</u>: **nabi chakra**, and press your body towards your legs. Do not stay here; instead, flow with your next *inhalation* straight into the next posture.

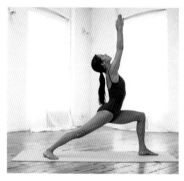

11 VIRABHADRASANA 1 (warrior 1) *Inhale* and repeat as for step 7, reversing your feet, so that you pivot your right foot to 45 degrees and step your left foot forwards in between your hands.

Moderation If your back heel rises off the floor and your hips swing open out of alignment, lessen the bend of your front leg.

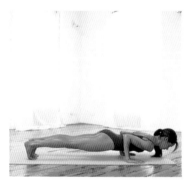

12 CHATURANGA DANDASANA (four limbs staff posture) *Exhale* and place your hands on either side of your left foot and take your left foot back by the right, lowering your body straight to the floor, <u>dristi</u>: **nasagrai.**

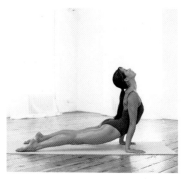

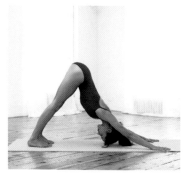

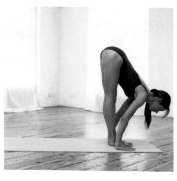

13 URDHVA MUKHA SVANASANA, (upward facing dog posture) *Inhale*, roll your shoulders back, lift up through your heart and arch your spine.

14 ADHO MUKHA SVANASANA (downward facing dog posture) *Exhale*, roll over your toes and send your hips back and up. *Take five long, slow, deep ujjayi breaths*, working deeply into the pose by pressing your chest open and connecting the tops of your arms into their shoulder sockets. Slide the shoulder blades up away from the ground, and lift your thigh muscles, abdomen and hips, while spreading your fingers and toes open into the floor. Look towards your navel, <u>dristi</u>: **nabi chakra**.

15 *Inhale* and jump into **URDHVA UTTANASANA** (upward intense stretch posture).

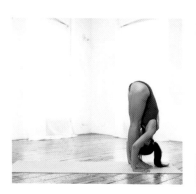

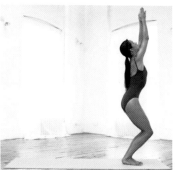

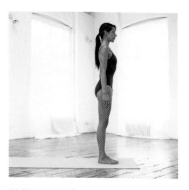

16 UTTANASANA (intense stretch posture) *Exhale* and fold your torso down towards your legs.

17 UTKATASANA (powerful posture) *Inhale* as you bend your knees and sink your hips low, lifting up through your abdomen and back and raising your arms sideways to bring your palms together (see step 1).

18 TADASANA (mountain posture) *Exhale* and gently press your palms downwards as you lower your arms down by the sides of your body. Feel your spine lengthening as you straighten your legs, and press the soles of your feet into the floor beneath you to return to Tadasana. Repeat Surya Namaskara B five to eight times.

Pādāṅguṣṭhāsana | FOOT BIG TOE POSTURE

pada = foot or leg
angustha = big toe

This posture teaches the basic mechanics of forward bending from deep within the hips, rather than from the lumbar region. Within this asana, the pelvis is tilted forwards and rotated over the tops of the thigh bones, and the torso is folded over the legs.

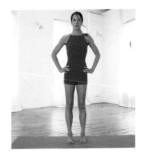

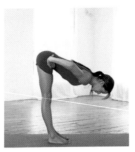

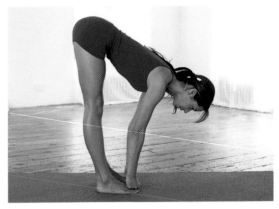

1 From Tadasana, *inhale* while softly jumping your feet slightly apart in line with your hips, aligning your knees to face the same direction as your toes. Sink your heels, big toe joints and outer edges of your feet deeply into the floor. Place your hands on your hips, relax your shoulders down, draw your thighs and lower abdomen up and lengthen your spine.

2 *Exhale slowly*, pivoting your pelvis forwards, and fold from your hips to extend your spine and torso out and over your legs.

3 *Inhale slowly* and catch hold of your big toes. Extend the crown of your head forwards and draw in your abdominal muscles to create length through your spine. Lift your thigh muscles and sitting bones. Root down into your feet while drawing your shoulders down your back and opening your collarbones wide.

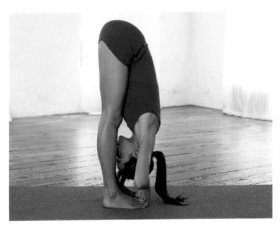

4 *Exhale slowly*, tilting your pelvis further forwards and bending deeper from your hips. Draw your head down and your body close in to your legs. Take your elbows out. Allow your shoulders to release up and away from the floor while lengthening the back of your neck. *Take five deep, slow ujjayi breaths*, allowing your back to yield to gravity. Draw in your abdominal muscles, float your sitting bones and extend your front ribs down. Lift your thigh muscles up and on to their bones. Move your chin in, relax the back of your neck and focus on your nose tip, <u>dristi</u>: **nasagrai**. *Inhale*, look up as in step 3 and lengthen your back. Go directly into Pada Hastasana or return to Tadasana, then perform steps 1–3 of Padangusthasana before moving on to Pada Hastasana.

Easing into the pose

Feeling strain, tension or pain is an indication of pushing too hard or of injury. Care must be taken for both. Remember to listen to your body: if you are unable to touch your toes, don't force it. To start with, try practising this pose by holding your ankles instead of your toes, slightly bending your knees. As you tilt your pelvis forwards release your hips over your legs.

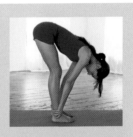

In time, the muscles in your back and legs will gradually become supple enough for you to reach your feet without bending your knees. Practise with patience, and you will be successful.

Deepening the pose

Each time you exhale, feel gravity pouring down through your spine, releasing your back out and down from your hips, while you softly press your buttocks higher and your heels deeper into the floor. Spread your toes open, pressing your big toes down firmly on to your first two fingers. Be lively in the arches of your feet.

Pāda Hastāsana | FOOT HAND POSTURE

pada = foot or leg
hasta = hand

This deepens the stretch of the previous asana, creating release and flexibility in the hips and legs. As the torso is drawn closer into the thighs, focus must be made on lengthening through the front of the torso to help prevent the back rounding over.

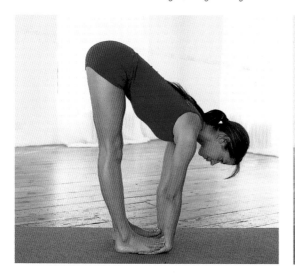

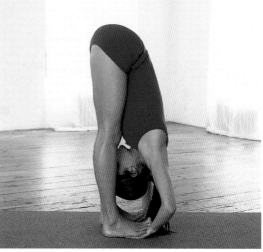

1 *Slowly exhale* and place your hands, palms upwards, under the soles of your feet. *Inhale* here and stretch your spine long deeply engaging uddiyana.

2 *Slowly exhale*. Hinge from your pelvis to fold your torso down and in towards your legs. Release your neck muscles to allow gravity to flow down through the entire length of your spine as the crown of your head descends. Press the back of your thighs and hips up, drawing uddiyana bandha deeper into your body. *Take five deep breaths*. Broaden across the back of your shoulders and keep your neck long. Open and spread the soles of your feet deeply into the palms of your hands, while sending your sitting bones up and the top of your skull down. Look along your nose tip, <u>**dristi: nasagrai**</u>. *Inhale* and lift your head as in step 1. *Exhale* and place your hands on your hips. *Inhale* and come up to a standing position. *Exhale* and softly jump your feet together to return to Tadasana.

Easing into the pose

If you cannot reach your feet yet, or if your back feels strained when you try, bend your knees, bringing your front ribs on to your thighs. Take your hands on to the floor if standing on them is uncomfortable. From here, gently begin to straighten your legs.

Alternatively, if you are suffering from spinal injuries or a prolapsed disc, stand facing a wall, a little way away from it. Extend your back forwards, lengthening it flat and forming a right angle with your legs. Stretch your arms out straight and press your palms open into the wall. Stay in this position, breathing length into your spine and legs for five breaths.

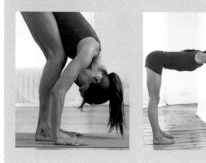

Deepening the pose

To intensify the stretch through the backs of the thighs (the hamstring muscles), press your weight through the balls of your feet into the palms of your hands. Gently draw the outer sides of your knees back to create good alignment; this will keep your knees correctly in line with your toes, which is

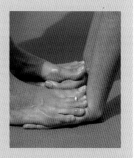

essential for healthy knees and legs.

Utthita Trikoṇāsana | EXTENDED TRIANGLE POSTURE

utthita = extended
tri = three
kona = angle

This posture draws energy up through the legs into the sideways stretch of the back. Strength and flexibility are developed in the feet, ankles, legs and hips, creating a secure foundation for all the following wide-legged asanas.

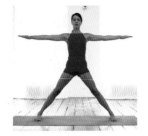
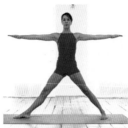

1 From Tadasana, *inhale* and softly jump (or step) to the right, so that you face to the side of your yoga mat, taking your feet about 110cm/45in apart. Keep your legs strong and lift your kneecaps and thigh muscles up. Open the soles of your feet, pressing them down into the ground and aligning them completely parallel to one another. Stretch your arms open and out to the sides in line with your shoulders. Feel your back gently extending up and your shoulders releasing down. Keep your chin level.

2 Begin a *long, slow exhalation*, and turn your left leg, toes and ball of the foot inwards by 10–15 degrees, while turning your right leg outwards by 90 degrees. Place your right heel opposite your left arch, and keep your hips level and your tailbone releasing downwards. Remember to keep your knees aligned over your toes, so that the turning rotation of your legs occur within your hip sockets.

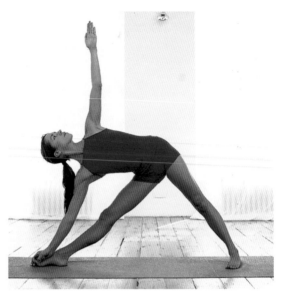

3 Continue to *exhale slowly*, and stretch your torso out to the right side over your right leg. Do not lean forwards as you catch hold of your right big toe. Draw your left hip back and outwards. Stretch your left arm up with the hand directly over your left shoulder lengthening through to your fingertips, with the palm facing forwards. Look towards your left hand, <u>dristi</u>: **hastagrai**. *Take five to ten long, steady breaths*, opening your body out like a star. With a *slow inhalation*, draw your body upright, turning your feet parallel. *Exhale slowly*, and repeat step 2, this time turning your right leg in by 10–15 degrees and your left leg out by 90 degrees and stretch over to the left side. *Take five to ten deep, slow breaths*, then *inhale* and draw your body upright, turning your feet parallel. From here, either go directly into the next posture or *exhale* and return to Tadasana. Then jump your feet apart and continue on to Parivrtta Trikonasana.

Easing into the pose
If your torso and hips lean forwards, the benefits of the lateral stretch to the torso will be lost. Instead of trying to grasp your toe, place your right hand lightly on your right shin or ankle instead, or on a wooden yoga block if you have one. Do not abandon the integrity of your practice for the pride of the pose. Work truthfully, and your suppleness will develop, allowing you to catch hold of your big toe in time.

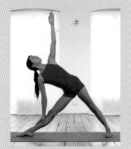
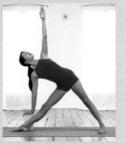

Deepening the pose
Work to draw your left hip back, gently moving the left ribs and shoulder directly over the right ribs and shoulder. Extending your left arm back and taking your fingertips on to your right upper thigh will help in sensing this side stretch.

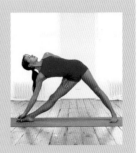

Parivṛtta Trikoṇāsana | REVOLVED TRIANGLE POSTURE

parivrtta = revolved, turned
tri = three
kona = angle

This posture creates a counter-stretch to Trikonasana and introduces the mechanics of twisting, which is essential for spinal health. To twist effectively, the legs and hips have to be firm while the twisting motion flows up through the spine to the head.

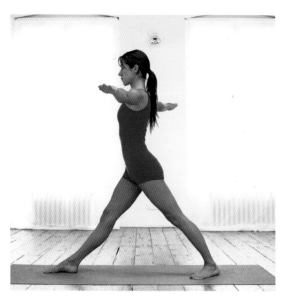

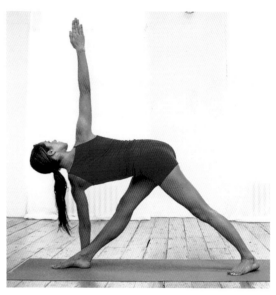

1 Begin to *exhale very slowly*, and turn your left toes, ball of foot, leg and hip in by 45 degrees while rotating your right hip, leg and foot out by 90 degrees. Turn your body to face completely to the right side, squaring both hip bones, collarbones and shoulders evenly, like sets of headlights all shining in the same direction. Stretch your arms out to the sides at shoulder height, and align your feet with their respective hips.

2 Continue to *exhale slowly*, and gently sweep your left arm and the left side of your torso forwards and down towards your right leg. Cross your left wrist over your right ankle, and open your left palm down on to the floor by the little-toe edge of your right foot. Revolve your right shoulder and the side of your right torso back. Extend your right arm up and over your right shoulder. Softly draw both shoulders down away from your ears, keeping your legs active (kneecaps and thigh muscles lifted) and your bandhas engaged. *Take five to ten breaths*, lifting and opening your chest skywards and looking towards your raised hand, <u>dristi</u>: **hastagrai**. With *an inhalation*, lift your torso up, turning your feet parallel, then *exhale* and repeat the pose to the left. *Take five to ten deep, smooth breaths*, then *inhale* and draw your torso upright, turning your feet parallel. *Exhale* and jump into Tadasana.

Easing into the pose
If your hand cannot reach the floor at first, rest it on your shin or ankle or a wooden yoga block, and work the rotation of your torso from here, taking the lifted hand on to the sacrum. With practice, the hand will gradually be able to touch the floor.

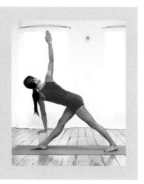

Deepening the pose
The stability of this posture is developed by the rootings of your feet into the ground. Open the sole of your back foot and outer heel deeply into the floor. Draw the muscles of your front thigh up and move your front hip back and your back hip forwards to balance your pelvis. Deepen the twist in the back by opening your right collarbone away from the left. Roll the right side of your torso up and back to align directly over the left side of your torso. On the second side to the posture, focus on drawing the left side of your torso over your right side.

Utthita Pārśvakoṇāsana | EXTENDED LATERAL ANGLE POSTURE

utthita = extended
parsva = side or lateral
kona = angle

This posture furthers the fundamental principles of Utthita Trikonasana with an extended side stretch. The deep lunging in one leg and the stretch through the other creates a dynamic balance of leg strength and flexibility.

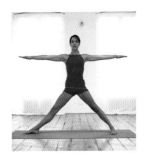 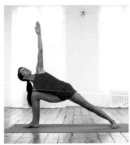 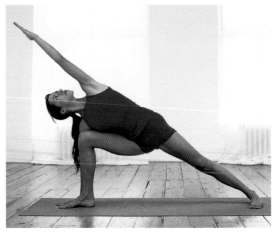

1 From Tadasana, *inhale* and softly jump (or step) to the right, taking your feet parallel and about 140cm/55in apart, with your arms extending out to the sides. Feel your legs stretching long and your spine lengthening up. Begin to *exhale very slowly*, turning your left foot and leg in by 15 degrees and rotating your right leg and foot out by 90 degrees (as in Utthita Trikonasana, step 2), and align your right heel opposite your left arch.

2 Continue to *exhale slowly*, and deeply bend your right knee, drawing the back of the knee completely over (but not beyond) your ankle to create a right angle through the right leg. Lengthen your body over to the right side, taking your right hand on to the floor by the little-toe edge of your right foot. Raise your left arm and extend it up over your shoulder.

3 As you complete your *exhalation*, soften your left shoulder down and rotate your left arm within its socket, then stretch the arm diagonally over by the side of your head, with the palm facing down. Look up towards the little-finger edge of your raised hand, **dristi: hastagrai**, and *take five to ten even, deep breaths*, drawing the entire length of the left side of your torso up and open to turn your chest skywards. *Inhale slowly*, straightening your knee and lifting your torso upright. Turn your feet parallel, then repeat Parsvakonasana to the left side. *Take five to ten deep, slow breaths*, then *inhale very slowly*, drawing your body upright and turning your feet parallel. From here, either go directly into Parivrtta Parsvakonasana as you begin your next *exhalation*, or *exhale* and lightly jump back into Tadasana. From here, *inhale* and lightly jump your feet 140cm/55in apart to the right, with the arms stretching to the sides at shoulder level, then continue on into Parivrtta Parsvakonasana with the next *exhalation*.

Easing into the pose
This posture creates a very deep and challenging stretch. If reaching for the floor causes your torso to lean forwards, avoid this by bending your elbow and placing your forearm on your thigh. This will also help in keeping the pelvis and hips open, your chest lifted and your waist

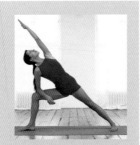

toned. You will gradually advance into the full posture.

Deepening the pose
Work your legs evenly and stretch them away from one another to create a balance of energy in the posture. Feel the legs releasing out from the pelvis and inner groin, then press your right knee and outer thigh back into the right arm, while stretching down through your left leg into left outer heel and little toe. (Reverse for other side.)

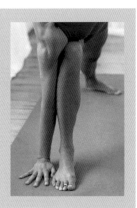

Parivṛtta Pārśvakoṇāsana | REVOLVED LATERAL ANGLE POSTURE

parivrtta = revolved, turned
parsva = side or lateral
kona = angle

In this strong twist, the ribcage is fully rotated, deepening the breath and improving respiration. As the torso is turned blood circulation is stimulated to the internal organs flushing them of toxins and boosting digestion. Leg strength is developed.

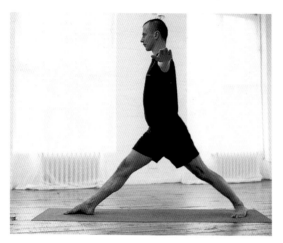

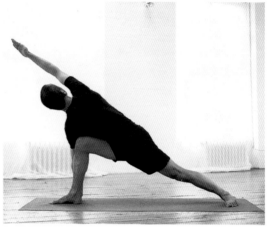

1 Begin to *exhale very slowly* as you rotate your left toes, ball of foot, leg and hip in by 45 degrees, and rotate your right hip, leg and foot out by 90 degrees (as in Parivrtta Trikonasana). Turn your body to face the right side, squaring your shoulders and hip bones evenly while stretching your arms out to the sides at shoulder height. Align your feet with their respective hip sockets.

2 Continue to *exhale slowly* and bend your right knee fully, taking it directly over your right ankle into a right angle. Turn your torso towards your right leg, drawing the left side of your ribcage over your right thigh. Extend your left armpit and arm over the outer side of your right knee and shin. Place your left hand on the floor by the outer side of your right foot. Revolve the right shoulder and side of your body back and up. Rotate your right arm within its shoulder socket to turn your palm to face over head, and stretch your arm diagonally over by the side of your head. Softly draw your shoulders down and press your chest open upwards as you root your back foot down. *Take five to ten breaths*, and look towards your raised hand along the outer edge, <u>dristi</u>: **hastagrai**. With a *slow inhalation*, return your torso upright and straighten your right leg, turning your feet parallel. Start to *exhale slowly*, and repeat steps 1 and 2, with the body turning to the left. *Exhale*, softly jump back into Tadasana.

Easing into the pose
This is a strong posture. If you feel any straining or twisting in your back knee, release the heel off the floor and let the knee touch down to the floor. Alternatively, if the knee feels strong but the chest caves in or the shoulders hunch up, work the back heel down into the floor, and hook your elbow

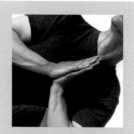

over the opposite thigh, then bring your palms together at the centre of your chest.

Deepening the pose
Cross your arm and shoulder completely over the opposite thigh. Focus on pressing the outer side of your knee and shin against the outer side of your shoulder and arm to help secure this powerful rotation of your torso. As you move into this pose, be sure to stretch the spine while opening the chest upwards.

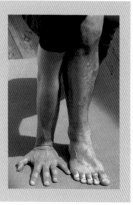

Prasārita Pādōttānāsana A | EXPANDED LEG STRETCH POSTURE A

prasarita = expanded or spread
pada = foot or leg
uttana = extended or intense
stretch

The four variations of this posture each work deeply on strengthening and stretching the legs, and the four work together to stimulate and cleanse the digestive organs. The first pose opens the hip joints and allows energy to flow from the pelvis to the feet.

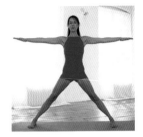

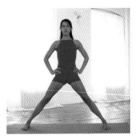

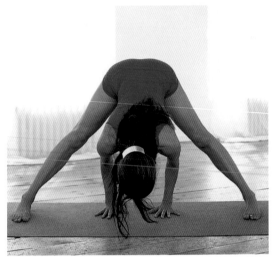

1 From Tadasana, *inhale* and softly jump (or step) to the right, taking your feet parallel and about 140cm/55in apart, with your arms lengthening out to the sides. Take your feet wide to align them directly under your wrists, with your arches strongly lifted.

2 *Exhale slowly*, opening the soles of your feet down into the floor, and place your hands on your hips. *Inhale slowly* and lengthen up through your spine, breathing openness into your back and pelvis. Draw your thigh muscles up, and be especially aware of uddiyana bandha now and throughout this whole series of the four Prasarita Padottanasanas.

3 *Exhale slowly* and extend your back forwards, folding deeply from your hips. Place your hands on the ground, in between your feet if possible. Spread your fingers and look at your hands, checking that they are shoulder-width apart and that your middle fingers are extending forwards. Keep your chest open and your shoulders relaxed.

Easing into the pose
If you experience strain in your back or over-pulling through the hamstring muscles, you can practise by bending your knees directly over your toes and placing your hands on the floor in line with your shoulders. Using yoga blocks or a pile of books can also be helpful, and in this way you can begin to work your legs straight without causing stress in your back.

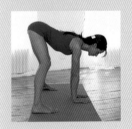

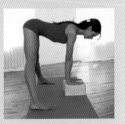

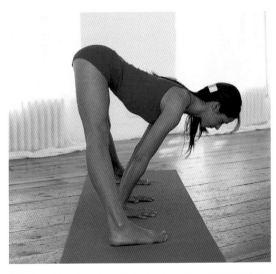

Deepening the pose
Spreading and opening your hands and feet into the floor will create a firm anchor for you, so that you can strongly float your sitting bones upwards. This will begin to increase the flexibility in your hips and legs. Keep long in your neck and open in your shoulders, releasing them up from the floor.

4 *Inhale* and lengthen through the front and back of your spine, drawing your chest and focus forwards while keeping your neck long and in line with your spine. Release your shoulder blades down your back and firmly lift your thigh muscles up.

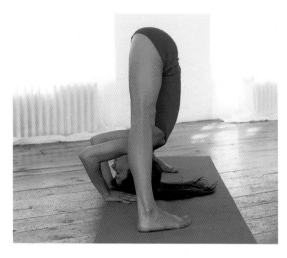

5 *Exhale slowly* into the full posture by pivoting your pelvis further forwards to deepen the rotation within your hip sockets. Step your hands back, so that your fingertips are in line with the heels of your feet, and lower the top of your head to the floor. Bend your elbows over your wrists and slide your shoulders up away from the floor. *Take five to ten slow, even breaths*, yielding your back to gravity, while keeping your legs strong and active by drawing up your thigh muscles. Move the skin of the outer edges of your knees back to prevent your knees misaligning or locking. Look to your nose tip, <u>dristi</u>: **nasagrai**, and open the soles of your feet. *Slowly inhale* and lift your focus and chest forwards. *Exhale*, extend your back flat and parallel to the floor, hands on your hips. *Inhale* and lift your torso up to standing position. From here, either move into posture B, or *exhale*, and jump back into Tadasana. Then *inhale*, jump to the right, parting your feet wide, and continue on to the B variation.

Prasārita Pādōttānāsana B | EXPANDED LEG STRETCH POSTURE B

prasarita = expanded or spread
pada = foot or leg
uttana = extended or intense
stretch

In this variation, the hands remain on the hips, allowing the spine to cascade forwards freely without pulling through the arms to draw the body low. This releases compression on the vertebrae, creating space in the spine and replenishing the inter-vertebral discs.

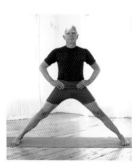

1 *Exhale* and, with your hands on your hips, feel your feet connecting down into the floor while drawing your thigh muscles up. *Inhale*, breathing length into your spine and openness into your chest and collarbones.

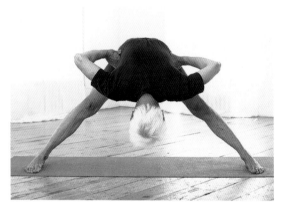

Easing into the pose
If your back rounds, bend your knees to help develop straightness and length through your spine and to facilitate a deeper pivoting of your pelvis forwards.

Deepening the pose
Be careful not to strain or push in this posture: as with all postures, suppleness comes not from straining but from releasing. Keeping this in mind each time you breathe out, feel gravity streaming down through your spine, helping to release your back and head lower. Do not allow your shoulders to press down to your ears; instead, gently slide them up and away.

2 *Exhale* and slowly fold your torso down by pivoting your pelvis forwards. Lengthen through your spine and extend the crown of your head to the floor. Keep your hands on your hips and *take five to ten deep, slow breaths*, again focusing on the dynamic energy in your legs. Be careful not to lock your knees; instead, gently but firmly press your inner thigh muscles away from one another. Look along to your nose tip, <u>dristi</u>: **nasagrai**. *Inhale* and lift from your abdominal muscles to return your torso up to standing position. *Exhale*, relax your shoulders and deepen uddiyana bandha. *Inhale* and lengthen your arms out to the sides at shoulder level. From here, either move straight into posture C, or *exhale* and lightly jump back into Tadasana. From Tadasana *inhale* and jump to the side, taking your feet wide apart and your arms open, then continue into posture C.

Prasārita Pādōttānāsana C | EXPANDED LEG STRETCH POSTURE C

prasarita = expanded or spread
pada = foot or leg
uttana = extended or intense
stretch

This posture creates an intense joint-opening stretch in the hips and legs and through the shoulders and arms. Creating a full rotation inside the shoulder sockets helps to loosen and prevent stiffness in the arms, shoulder girdle and upper back.

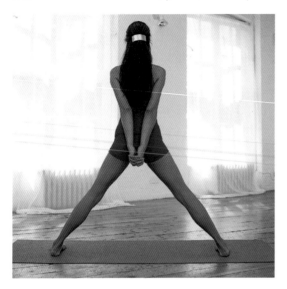

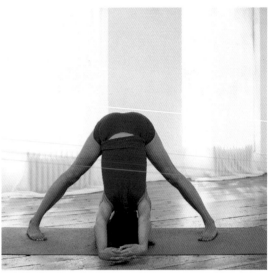

1 *Exhale*, take your hands behind your back and interlace your fingers. *Inhale*, draw your shoulders back and lengthen through your arms, rotating your inner arms forwards. Gently press your knuckles down and open across your chest and collarbones.

2 *Exhale slowly* and fold forwards from your hips, drawing your arms up and over behind your shoulders. Expand your chest, stretching your arms long and directing your little fingers down towards the floor. Feel your shoulder blades drawing inwards and allow your arms to rotate softly within their shoulder sockets. *Breathe* into the posture for *five to ten slow breaths*, looking along to your nose tip, <u>dristi</u>: **nasagrai**. *Inhale*, draw your abdominal muscles in to move your back upright, then draw your arms down behind your back. *Exhale* here relaxing your shoulders. *Inhale*, release the interlace of your fingers and stretch your arms out to the sides at shoulder level. From here, you can either flow into posture D as you begin your next *exhalation* or you can *exhale* and lightly jump back into Tadasana. From Tadasana *inhale* and jump to the right side, parting your feet wide, and then continue into the final variation of this posture.

Benefits of the pose
The muscles between the upper spine and shoulder blades (intraspinatus) are strengthened by this posture, as circulation to this region is stimulated. The chest and front ribs are expanded, improving respiration and helping to maintain the openness of the front torso.

Easing into the pose
As well as developing flexibility in your legs and hips, this variation creates suppleness in the shoulders and arms. If either your shoulders or arms, or both, feel unable to yield, use a belt or yoga strap to link your hands and then gently work to extend your arms over and you can still benefit. Keep moving your

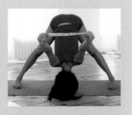

shoulder blades in at the same time as drawing the shoulders back, as this will release tension from the shoulder girdle.

Deepening the pose
Softly move your chin in to bring length to the back of your neck. This also creates space for the rotation and movement of your shoulders needed to release your arms over. Press down through your heels while firmly lifting your front thigh muscles up and on to your thigh bones. Keep your feet active and lift your arches.

prasarita = expanded or spread
pada = foot or leg
uttana = extended or intense
stretch

The final variation of Prasarita Padottanasana strongly stimulates the digestive fire (agni), thereby aiding the digestive process and internal cleansing. The space created between the shoulder blades opens the pathway through the spine into the brain.

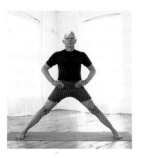
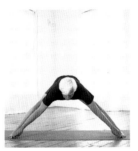

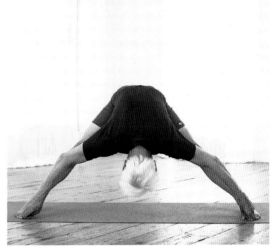

1 *Exhale slowly* and place your hands on your hips while opening the soles of your feet down into the floor. *Inhale slowly*, keeping your hands on your hips, and lengthen up through your spine. Breathe openness into your chest and collarbones as you focus on drawing your thigh muscles up on to the thighbones. Fully engage uddiyana bandha.

2 *Exhale slowly* and extend your back forwards, folding deeply at the hips. Catch hold of your big toes using the index and middle fingers of both hands as in Padangusthasana (foot big toe posture page 50). *Inhale* and lengthen through your spine, drawing your chest and focus out and forwards. Extend your back long, keeping your neck in line with your spine, and stretch the front of your torso. Move your shoulder blades down your back away from your ears, and firmly lift your thighs.

3 *Exhale slowly*, bending your elbows outwards and hinging deeper within your hip sockets. Release your neck muscles to allow the top of your head to drop towards the floor. Feel the flow of gravity moving down through your spine. Soften your shoulders wide in the same direction as your elbows, and be careful to slide your shoulder blades up and away from your ears. *Take five to ten steady, even breaths*, looking along to your nose tip, **dristi: nasagrai**. *Slowly inhale*, lengthening your spine and lifting your focus and chest forwards, while keeping the back of your neck long. With your fingers still holding your toes, straighten your arms as in step 2. *Exhale* and place your hands on your hips. Extend your back long, stretching the front of your torso parallel to the floor. *Inhale*, lifting up from your abdominal muscles, and draw your torso up to standing position, while opening the soles of your feet down into the floor. *Exhale* and lightly jump your feet together into Tadasana, facing the front of your mat.

Easing into the pose

Bend your knees to release any strain or pressure in your back, and hold your ankles if you are initially unable to take hold of your big toes.

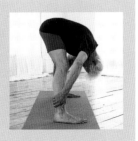

Deepening the pose

Soften the fold at the front of your hips and focus on sending your tailbone, sitting bones and pubic bone back and up to release your spine, and the crown of your head down towards the floor. Keep your legs active, and strongly press your inner thighs away from one another, extending energy down through to the soles of your feet into the floor. Work uddiyana bandha throughout these four poses to increase the benefits and to support and protect the back.

Pārśvōttānāsana | SIDE INTENSE STRETCH POSTURE

parsva = side or lateral
uttana = extended or intense
stretch

This posture develops the alignment, symmetry and balance of the pelvis and hips while strengthening the leg muscles. It stimulates circulation, deepens breathing, improves posture – especially hunching of the back – and unlocks tension.

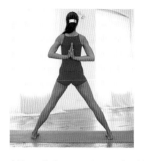

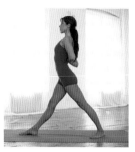

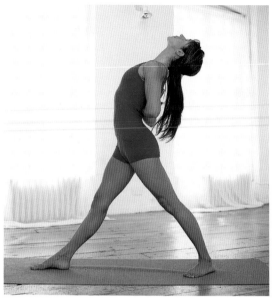

1 From Tadasana, *inhale* and softly jump (or step) to the right, taking your feet about 110cm/45in apart, and open your arms out to the sides in line with your shoulders. Open the soles of your feet and align them parallel to one another. Feel your back gently extending up and your shoulders releasing down. Begin to *exhale slowly* and draw your palms together behind your back into a prayer gesture (*paschima namaste*).

2 Continue to *exhale* and turn your left toes, ball of foot, leg and hip in by 45 degrees, while rotating your right hip, leg and foot out by 90 degrees. Turn your body to face completely to the right side, squaring both hip bones, collarbones and shoulders.

3 *Inhale* and roll your shoulders back and down. Raising your focus and heart, look up, while pressing your palms together.

Easing into the pose
If taking your palms together into paschima namaste is not yet possible, hold your elbows behind your back. Gradually your shoulder flexibility will develop so your hands can come together.

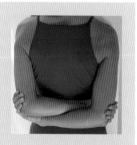

Deepening the pose
In the full posture, roll your elbows backwards and draw your shoulder blades in, to create an openness in your heart and chest. The legs and hips need to be correctly aligned to gain the full benefits of this posture. Focus on strongly drawing

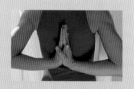

your front kneecap and thigh muscle up to the right hip, while pressing the ball of your front foot down.

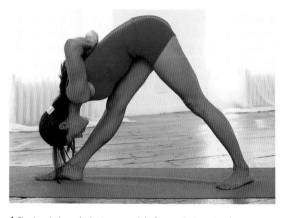

4 *Slowly exhale* and pivot your pelvis forwards to extend your torso out and over your right leg, bringing your face towards your shin. As you *take five to ten deep, even breaths*, elongate the front and back of your spine and lengthen through the back of the neck, releasing your head down. Focus your gaze towards your nose tip, **dristi: nasagrai**. With a *slow inhalation*, lift from uddiyana bandha, returning your torso upright and bringing your feet parallel. Repeat steps 2–4 turning to the left. *Exhale* and softly jump into Tadasana, releasing the arms down.

utthita = extended
hasta = hand
pada = foot or leg
angustha = big toe

This and the three following extended postures flow consecutively into one another creating dynamic power in the muscles of the supporting leg to maintain the balance effectively for the duration of these four asana variations.

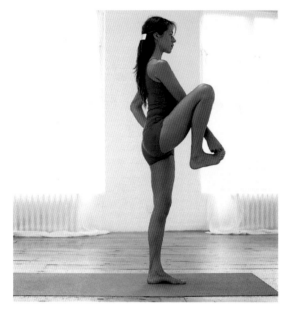

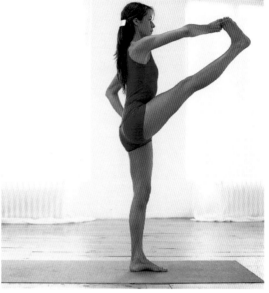

1 From Tadasana, *inhale*, gently swing your right knee up, and, using your right index and middle fingers, catch hold of your right big toe. Press your right big toe into your fingers and draw your right hip down to keep it level with the left. Place your left hand on to your left hip, and balance.

2 With a *slow, steady exhalation*, press your right foot up, lengthening your leg straight and up towards your chest. Release the front of your right hip down, creating a seesaw action to raise your right foot and shinbone higher. Roll both your shoulders back and down, and bend your right elbow outwards to help keep your chest open. *Breathe steadily here*, connecting uddiyana bandha deeply into your body, and align your lifted foot directly forwards. Gaze steadily to your right toes, <u>**dristi: padhayoragrai**</u>. *After five to ten full breaths, inhale*, straighten your right arm and flow into the next posture.

Easing into the pose
If straightening your leg causes your back to round and your shoulders to hunch, practise this posture at first with your knee bent, as in step 1. With each practice, press your lifted foot slightly forwards to gradually stretch your hamstring. Over time and with practice, you will develop both the strength and flexibility to lengthen the leg straight without compromising the alignment of your back.

Deepening the pose
Do not over-focus on your raised leg: it is really your standing foot and leg that deserve your awareness, since they create your base and support in this posture. Consciously stretch your standing leg, rooting the sole of your open foot into the floor and drawing your knee and thigh up. Focus on aligning the knee and toes forwards and keep the right

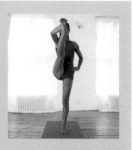

side of your right hip softening down level with the left hip. Press your lifted heel directly forwards.

Utthita Pārśvasahita A | EXTENDED SIDE ACCOMPANIED POSTURE A

utthita = extended
parsva = side or lateral
sahita = accompanied

Opening the raised leg to the side in this asana further enhances balance, co-ordination and mental concentration. Keeping the back straight develops the strength of the muscles on either side of the spine. The legs and buttocks are also toned.

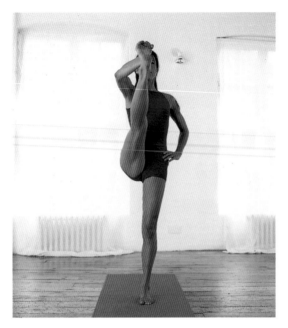

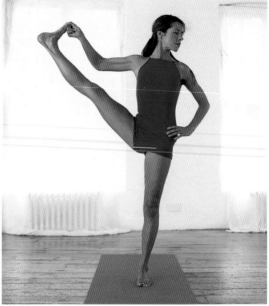

1 From the previous posture as pictured above, take a *long, even exhalation*, open your right arm and leg out to the right side, rotating your inner thigh forwards and releasing your right buttock and tailbone downwards. Open your chest and slide your shoulder blades down your back to create length through your spine and neck.

2 Turn your head to the left, moving your chin over your left shoulder, and *take five to ten breaths* here, levelling your collarbones open and extending your focus out to the right side, **dristi: parsva**. *Inhale*, and return your right arm, leg and focus forwards, then flow into the next posture.

Easing into the pose
As in the previous posture, you can work this pose with your leg bent, focusing on gradually lengthening and straightening it a little more with each practice. Be patient, and, with practice and a calm approach, the full posture will soon be achievable.

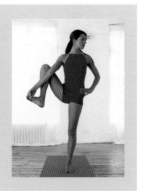

Deepening the pose
Feel the whole pose opening out from your centre in three flowing energy lines:
1 From the back of your waist upwards along your spine through to the very top of your head.
2 Down from the back of your waist through into your tailbone and standing leg, sending the sole of your foot deeper into the floor.
3 Out from the inner thigh of your raised leg through to the heel.
Breathe into these three energy lines and let the posture grow and expand.

utthita = extended
parsva = side or lateral
sahita = accompanied

This creates an amazing stretch through the legs and hips. Pressing down through the supporting leg and foot is crucial for stability. An awareness of gravity and the energy rising up through the body will help to centre and balance the mind and body.

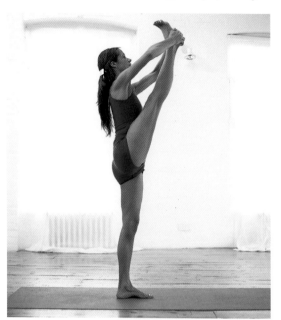

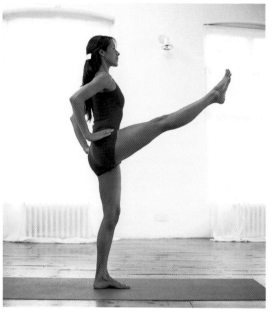

1 With a *smooth exhalation*, catch hold of your right foot with both hands. Root down through your standing foot to lift your raised foot higher. If your standing leg begins to feel weak or tired, focus on sending the energy of your breath down through to your foot, and open your foot into the floor to receive the energy pouring up into your muscles, providing them with strength and vitality. Do not straighten your arms, instead keep your elbows bent. *Take five to ten slow breaths*, looking towards your right toes, <u>dristi</u>: **padhayoragrai**, and then *exhale*, releasing the hold on your foot without dropping your foot to the floor.

2 With your hands on your hips, keep your leg lifted and float your foot to 90 degrees or higher without straining or hunching your back. *Take five full, steady breaths*, stretching up through your back and releasing your shoulders down. Softly gaze towards the toes of your right foot, <u>dristi</u>: **padhayoragrai**. *Exhale* and slowly lower the foot, returning to Tadasana. Repeat Utthita Hasta Padangusthasana, and Utthita Parsvasahita A and B/C on the left side.

Easing into the pose
Maintaining a length and energy flow through your spine is essential for spinal alignment and health. Yoga postures are intended to develop and enhance this energy and health, so do not at any time during your practice sacrifice length and alignment of your spine for the grandeur of a posture. There are no benefits to be gained by straining and hunching your back in an attempt to lift your leg high. In fact, it is more beneficial not to lift your leg so high, or practise initially with the lifted knee bent instead to maintain a strong, straight back. Practising in this way will gradually develop your strength, alignment and flexibility.

Deepening the pose
As you draw your right leg and your foot up, feel the opposite end of the same leg, i.e. the top of your thigh bone, connecting down into its hip socket. In this way, a seesaw motion is created, helping to float the lifted foot further up. Feel the right sitting bone drawing down in line with the left to keep the pelvis aligned. Open the sole of your standing foot deeply down into the ground.

Ardha Baddha Padmōttānāsana | HALF BOUND LOTUS INTENSE STRETCH

ardha = half
baddha = bound or caught
padma = lotus
uttana = extended/intense stretch

Here the beginnings of the lotus posture are introduced. In the full posture, the heel presses into the lower abdomen, stimulating blood circulation through the intestines. Strength is promoted through the standing leg, and the binding arm creates openness.

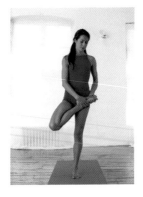
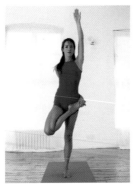

1 *Inhale*. Bend your right knee, lifting your foot up. Use both hands to place your foot at the very top of your left front thigh. Move the little-toe edge of your right foot up to the left hip socket, and gently direct the right kneecap downwards. This is half lotus.

2 Continue to *inhale*. Stretch your right arm behind your back and reach your right hand to your right foot, catching hold of the right big toe with your index and middle fingers. Release your left hand from your foot and stretch your left arm up. (If you need to steady your balance here, do so, and *breathe out and then in* as you raise your left arm; otherwise move directly on.)

3 *Exhale*, and extend your torso forwards, bending your left knee slightly, and softly fold your back down over your left leg. Place your left hand on the floor next to your left foot and keep your right hand holding your right big toe.

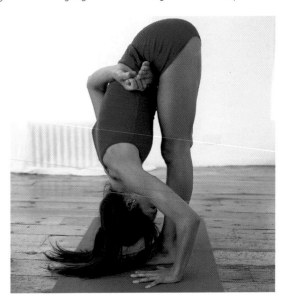

Inhale, breathing length into your spine, and softly roll your shoulders back and straighten your left leg. *Fully exhale*, and fold your torso deeply in towards your left leg, relaxing your neck muscles and releasing your head low. Move your face towards your left shin and *breathe steadily here for five to ten breaths*, looking towards the nose tip, <u>**dristi: nasagrai**</u>. *Inhale* and lift your chest forwards, then *exhale* and slightly bend your left knee. *Inhale* and lift from your abdominal muscles to bring your torso up to stand tall, straightening your left knee as you arrive upright. *Exhale* and release your right leg from the half lotus, then place your foot on the floor, returning to Tadasana. *Inhale*, lift the left foot into half lotus and repeat the posture on this side. After 5–10 breaths, *exhale* and return to Tadasana.

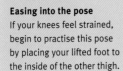
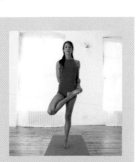

Easing into the pose
If your knees feel strained, begin to practise this pose by placing your lifted foot to the inside of the other thigh.

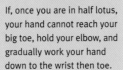

If, once you are in half lotus, your hand cannot reach your big toe, hold your elbow, and gradually work your hand down to the wrist then toe.

Deepening the pose
Press your lower abdomen towards your raised heel while drawing the thigh muscle of your standing leg firmly upwards. Broaden the sole of the standing foot strongly down to create a stable foundation. Once your balance is secure, try furthering the pose by

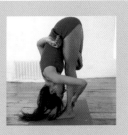

taking your hand off the floor and placing it on the back of your standing ankle.

Vinyasa into Utkaṭāsana | POWERFUL POSTURE

utkata = powerful or fierce or uneven

The following sequences create a wave of energy as the body flows through the sun salutations to link the last standing postures together through vinyasa. Utkatasana opens the knee joints and helps to remove ankle stiffness.

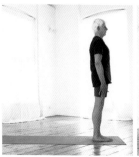

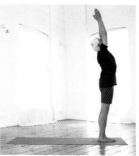

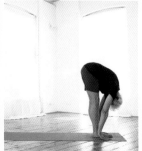

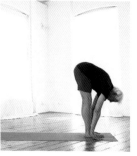

From Tadasana, flow through **Surya Namaskara A**, as follows.

—→ *Inhale*, drawing the breath deep into your lungs, and lift the arms into **Urdhva Tadasana** (upward mountain).

—→ *Exhale* and draw your body deep down to your legs into **Uttanasana** (intense stretch posture).

—→ *Inhale* and open your chest forwards into **Urdhva Uttanasana** (upwards intense stretch posture).

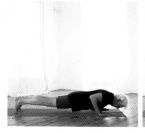

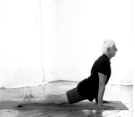

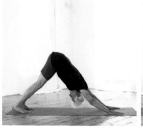

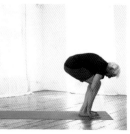

—→ *Exhale* and jump back into **Chaturanga Dandasana** (staff posture).

—→ *Inhale* and arch up into **Urdhva Mukha Svanasana** (upward facing dog), lifting your heart.

—→ *Exhale* and press your hips up into **Adho Mukha Svanasana** (downfacing dog) releasing your neck and head.

—→ *Inhale* and lightly jump your feet together in between your hands.

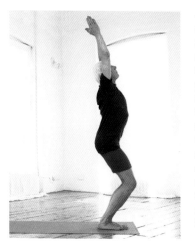

—→ *Continue to inhale* raising your arms up and deeply bending your knees. Fully engage uddiyana bandha and sink your hips and buttocks low. Stretch the sides of your waist up to your fingertips, creating a counter-balance to gravity. Bring your palms together overhead. Soften the fold at the back of your knees and in the front of your ankles to increase the depth of the posture. *Take five to ten deep, slow breaths,* drawing your focus softly up beyond your thumbs towards the sky, **dristi: urdhva**. From this posture of Utkatasana, move directly into a vinyasa, as overleaf.

Easing into the pose
If you feel tension in your shoulders, try parting your hands and taking your arms a little wider to make more room for your shoulders to drop. Slide your shoulder blades down, direct your focus down and lower your chin slightly towards your chest.

Vinyasa into Vīrabhadrāsana I | WARRIOR POSTURE I

Virabhadra = a warrior hero created from the hair of Siva, third god of the Hindu Trinity

There are three warrior postures, which are all dedicated to Virabhadra. The first two are practised here in the primary series and the third is introduced in the third series. They cultivate stamina, co-ordination and transitional smoothness of motion.

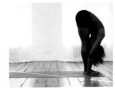 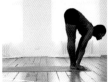 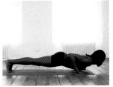 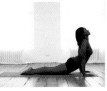 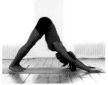

1 *Exhale* from the previous asana of Utkatasana and fold into **Uttanasana** (intense stretch).

⟶ *Inhale* and open your chest forwards into **Urdhva Uttanasana** (upwards intense stretch posture).

⟶ *Exhale* and jump back into **Chaturanga Dandasana** (staff posture).

⟶ *Inhale* and arch up into **Urdhva Mukha Svanasana** (upward facing dog posture), lifting your heart.

⟶ *Exhale*, press your hips up into **Adho Mukha Svanasana** (downward facing dog posture) and release your neck low.

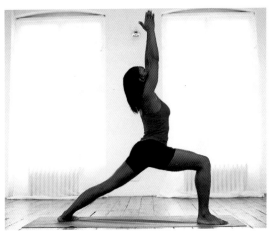

2 *Slowly inhale* and pivot on the ball of your left foot, rotating your heel inwards and forwards by 45 degrees towards your right arch. Step your right foot forwards in between your hands and align it with your right hip. Deeply bend your right knee, drawing it over the ankle, while pressing the sole of your left foot firmly into the floor. Bring your torso upright, opening your arms sideways and then up overhead with your palms together. Lift your face up and look towards your thumbs, <u>dristi:</u> **angustha ma dyai**. *Take five to ten breaths* in Virabhadrasana I.

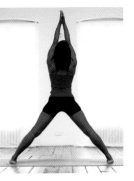 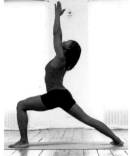

3 *Inhale*, straighten your right leg and turn your feet parallel to face the left side of your mat.

4 *Slowly exhale*, rotate your right toes, ball of foot, leg and hip in by 45 degrees, and turn your left hip, leg and foot out by 90 degrees, squaring your body to face the back edge of your yoga mat. Align your left foot with your left hip and deeply bend your left knee directly over the ankle into Virabhadrasana I. *Take five to ten long breaths* and then move on into Virabhadrasana II.

Easing into the pose

Keeping the hips equally aligned is of prime importance in this posture, so if you feel the hip of your back leg swinging backwards, decrease the bend in your front knee and focus on drawing your hip bone forwards. It can help to place your hands on your hips to steer them in the same direction. Keep the back foot firmly pushing down, especially the outer edge.

Deepening the pose

Allow your tailbone, hips and pelvis to release down with gravity, and feel your front thigh stretching long as your front knee draws forwards over the ankle to create a right angle (your shin vertical and your thigh parallel to the floor). Take care not to let the front knee fall inwards, and move the outer knee over your little toe. Lengthen both sides of your waist evenly, lifting your lower abdomen and raising your chest. Soften your shoulders down and let them align directly above and over your hips.

Vīrabhadrāsana II | WARRIOR POSTURE 2

Virabhadra = a warrior hero created from the hair of Shiva, third god of the Hindu trinity

Here, the hip joints are opened, releasing energy and blood circulation from the pelvis into the legs and increasing the muscular power of the lower body. The arms are toned and strengthened as they are drawn wide, helping to open the chest and ribcage.

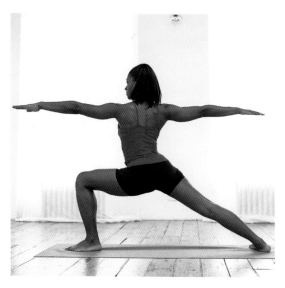

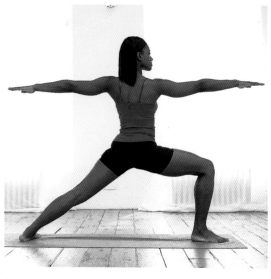

1 From Virabhadrasana I, maintain the deep bend of your left knee. *Exhale*, opening your arms wide out to the sides and stretching through to your fingertips at shoulder level. Draw your right hip bone and right collarbone open outwards away from the left. Align your feet so that your right foot is rotated in at a 15-degree angle and your left foot is open by 90 degrees, with the heel opposite the right arch, as in Parsvakonasana. *Take five to ten steady breaths*, breathing openness into your whole body and looking towards your left hand, <u>dristi</u>: hastagrai. *Inhale*, straighten your left leg, lengthen your spine and turn your feet parallel.

2 *Slowly exhale*, turn your feet (rotating your left foot inwards by 15 degrees and your right leg outwards by 90 degrees, with your right heel opposite your left arch), and bend your right knee over its own heel into a right angle, so repeating Virabhadrasana II to the right side. *Take another five to ten breaths*, this time looking over your right hand, <u>dristi</u>: hastagrai.

3 *Exhale* and place your hands on the floor. Step your right leg back, lowering into **Chaturanga Dandasana**.

⟶ *Inhale* into **Urdhva Mukha Svanasana**.

⟶ *Exhale* into **Adho Mukha Svanasana** and move straight to the jump through (overleaf).

Easing into the pose
The Virabhadrasana sequence challenges the strength of your legs, so be sure to breathe deeply to supply them with oxygen. If fully bending the knee causes the opposite foot to lose its connection with the floor, ease out of the bend slightly and re-root the opposite foot firmly down

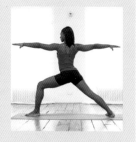

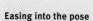

through the outer edge of the foot and heel.

Deepening the pose
Centre your torso directly over your pelvis, relax your shoulders and broaden your collarbones. Feel your legs opening wide and out from the pelvis, and move the pubic bone down to be at the same level as your bent knee. As always, pay attention to aligning the knees in the same direction as your toes and to rooting your feet.

Jump Through

The vinyasa into the jump through develops muscular and mental co-ordination while harnessing the power of the bandhas. This sequence of movement creates a transitional flow from standing to sitting, allowing your practice to become a continuous stream of flowing motion.

The vinyasa is based upon Surya Namaskara (sun salutation), the cornerstone of Astanga practice. The breath links each movement to create a flowing whole. This carries us through the sitting postures all the way through to the end of the practice. The vinyasa helps to maintain the internal body heat so that your muscles can yield and deeply stretch into the floor postures.

Learning the following jump through may take time, patience and practice, but it is integral to developing the fluidity of each vinyasa. It will also cultivate continuity of motion and build complete body and mind co-ordination, strength and a sense of flight while harnessing the power of the bandhas.

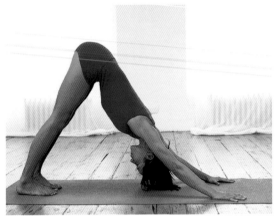

⟶ From exhaling into **Adho Mukha Svanasana** (downward facing dog posture), deeply engage uddiyana bandha.

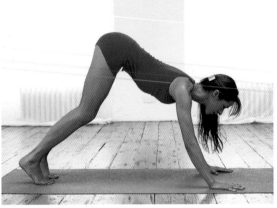

⟶ Continue to *exhale* as you shift your weight forwards on to your hands, letting your heels rise. Direct your focus at the space between your hands. Move your shoulders forwards and open your chest.

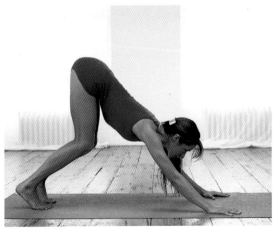

⟶ Bend your knees and take a gentle rebound back on to your feet. This will act as a springboard now for the jump/float through of your legs.

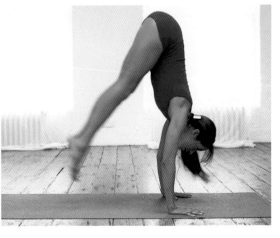

⟶ As you *inhale*, softly jump, moving your shoulders over your hands and swinging your hips in an arch over your shoulders. This will transfer all your weight and centre of balance into your hands, allowing your feet and legs to float up. Lift up out of your shoulders and press your palms down.

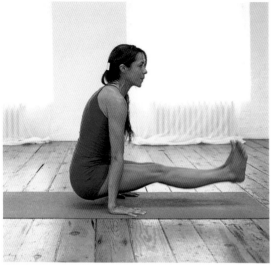

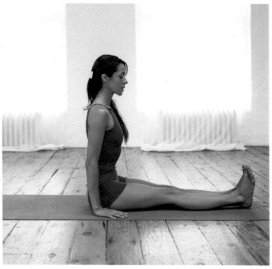

⟶ Continue to *inhale*, while keeping uddiyana bandha strong, and now swing your legs forwards through your arms, extending your feet out, and float your hips forwards. As soon as your legs start to descend, extend your focus forwards to and beyond your toes. Press your palms firmly down and lift your abdomen up to hover your hips, for a moment, just above the floor.

⟶ Keeping uddiyana bandha engaged, lower your buttocks completely down to sit. As your buttocks touch down, lift uddiyana bandha again. Lengthen your back and sit tall in **Dandasana** (staff posture). *Exhale.*

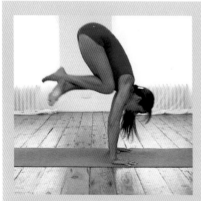

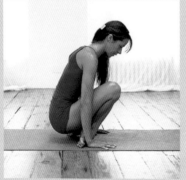

Easing into the pose
This vinyasa jump through may take much time and practice to perfect, so at first try as you jump to cross your ankles and tuck your knees up and into your chest. Press your palms strongly into the floor and lift your shoulders, to help find a moment of suspension before the legs start to lower.

Land softly on to the front of your feet just behind your hands. Roll back onto your buttocks and straighten your crossed legs into Dandasana. Once this becomes easy, slowly work towards swinging your legs straight through to land softly on your buttocks.

Deepening the pose
If you keep practising you will master this jump through. You will find that you can begin to focus on suspending your hips over your hands and finding a point of balance at the highest point of the jump up, that is just before beginning the descent. Engaging your bandhas is crucial, as this will create control and lightness in your pelvis, enabling you to suspend and balance here and helping you to develop a smooth, floating quality to your jump through.

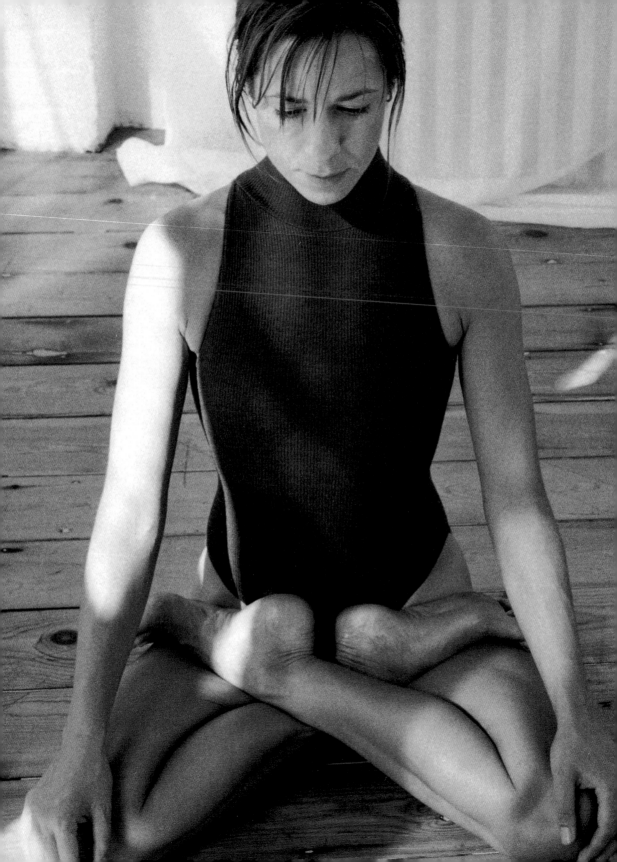

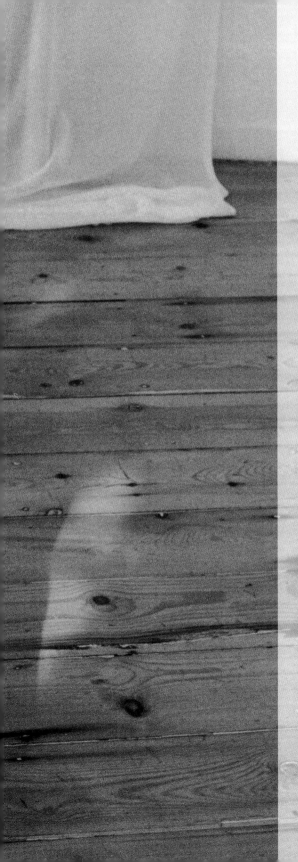

Seated Asanas

The seated asanas provide us with the chance to take the alignment and balance created in the standing sequence into a broader range of postures. The heat that has been generated will enable deep stretching, and the vinyasas between each side of each pose and each asana will help to maintain this internal heat.

The following seated postures, which form the central part of the primary series, purify the internal organs (including the heart) and the muscles while deeply articulating the joints of the body. They release physical, mental and emotional tensions and unlock energy to create physical strength, suppleness and openness of mind. Tightness and rigidity on all levels are challenged.

Focusing on the fullness of each breath will help you to move through these asanas and, as you do so, listen to all that arises within your mind and heart. In this way, we begin to cleanse the body and free the mind from past experiences, letting the breath wash through, bringing in new energy with each in-breath and releasing old energy with each out-breath.

By practising these asanas, a calmness of mind is brought about, an openness of heart and body is rediscovered and a secure connection with the ground is achieved.

Daṇḍāsana | STAFF POSTURE

danda = staff, rod or stick

This is the foundation from which all other seated asanas stem. Dandasana teaches us to sit in stillness. The subtle motion of breath flows through the limbs to bring this posture alive, activating and exercising every muscle of the body.

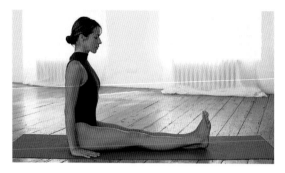

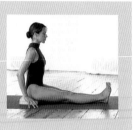

Easing into the pose
If you have tight hamstring muscles or any stiffness or injury in your back, practise this posture sitting on a yoga block or firm cushion to provide extra lift and support for your lower back.

Inhale, anchor your sitting bones into the floor, then lengthen from your lower spine to the crown of your head. Gently press your palms down and feel your shoulders descend. Lift your chest, keeping the back of your neck long, and open your collarbones. Focus on your nose tip, <u>dristi</u>: **nasagrai**, while fully engaging your bandhas to stretch your abdomen up. Press your heels away and draw the front thigh muscles upwards to your hips. Feel the backs of your legs long and open against the floor. *Take five to ten breaths*, then move into the next posture.

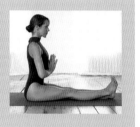

Deepening the pose
As your back gains strength, release your hands from the floor and bring them together in front of the chest in prayer position (namaste). Maintain the lift through the entire length of your spine.

Paschimottānāsana A/B/C/D | INTENSE STRETCH OF THE WEST A/B/C/D

paschima = west (which represents the back in yoga)
uttana = extended or intense stretch

This seated position allows the mechanics of the standing forward bends to be deepened as the torso rests down on the legs, developing flexibility and removing tension and stiffness. Each hand hold moves the body deeper into Paschimottanasana.

Paschimottanasana A

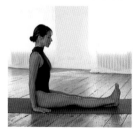

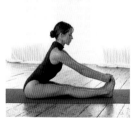

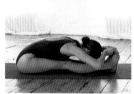

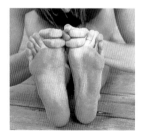

1 Start in Dandasana.

2 *Inhale* and raise your arms gently, extending your back forwards from your hips. Catch hold of your big toes, maintaining openness across your chest and length through the front and back of your spine and neck. Take care not to round your back or shorten the front of your body. Lifting the abdominal muscles (uddiyana bandha), opening your chest and rolling your shoulders back will help to prevent this collapse in the torso.

3 *Exhale* and pivot your pelvis forwards, folding your torso out and over your legs. Send your pubic bone back and down into the floor and lengthen your spine forwards. Feel your sitting bones anchoring down and the crown of your head floating towards your toes. Bend your elbows softly and slide your shoulder blades down your back. Lower your head but keep energy and focus extending out to your feet. *Take five deep breaths* in Paschimottanasana A, then *inhale*, draw your chest up, straighten your arms, and roll your shoulders back.

Paschimottanasana B

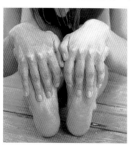

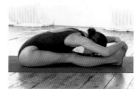

1 *Exhale* and change your hand position by taking your hands over your toes, pointing your fingertips towards your heels and pressing your palms and the soles of your feet together. *Inhale*, breathing length into your back.

2 *Exhale* and hinge deeply in the front of your hips, extending your chest further forwards towards your knees and drawing the elbows wide. This is Paschimottanasana B. Release tension in your neck and shoulders and allow your torso to surrender with gravity down over your legs. *After a full five even breaths, inhale* and draw your chest up, straightening your arms and lengthening your back diagonally forwards. Now continue into Paschimottanasana C.

Paschimottanasana C

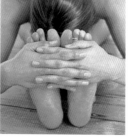

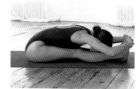

1 *Exhale*, release your hand position from the soles of your feet and interlock your fingers behind the balls of your feet. *Inhale*, lengthen your spine, look forwards and relax your shoulders.

2 *Exhale* and extend the front of your torso long, out and over your legs. Bring your chin on to your shins and move your forehead towards your ankles. Softly bend your elbows wide and focus on fully pivoting your pelvis forwards and deepening the fold in your hips. This is Paschimottanasana C. *Take five steady breaths* and, with your *sixth inhalation*, draw your chest up, lifting your head away from your legs and straightening your arms.

Paschimottanasana D

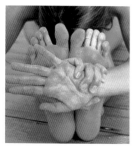

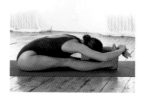

1 *Exhale*, release the interlock of your fingers and take the right hand to clasp your left wrist gently (or vice versa). *Inhale* as you extend your back long and lift your chest open.

2 *Exhale* and fold completely over your legs, sliding your pubis back and down and extending your breastbone forwards and out. Soften the back of your legs down into the floor and rest the entire length of your front torso on the front of your legs. Bend your elbows outwards and relax your shoulders. *Take five deep, slow breaths* in this final variation, Paschimottanasana D, then *inhale*, lifting your chest and head up.

• *Exhale*, release your hands from your feet and place your palms down just in front of your hips. From here, move into **jump back** and **vinyasas** as described overleaf.

Easing into the pose
A and B If you have back stiffness or pain, wrap a strap around the balls of your feet and take your hands as close as possible to your feet. Lengthen your back and keep your legs and feet together.
C and D If you need a strap to reach your feet, continue working as in posture A and focus on surrendering into the posture with each

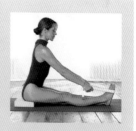

exhalation rather than forcing your torso down. If you are kind to your muscles, they will be more responsive and supple.

Deepening the pose
A and B Draw your lower abdominal muscles up and in. Work softly and deeply, and do not pull sharply on your arms or shoulders to increase the depth of the posture – this will cause either injury or tension, not flexibility.
C and D Draw the tops of your arms deep into their shoulder sockets and soften your shoulder blades down away from your ears. In all 4 asanas relax your neck muscles and lower your head while sending energy and focus out through the crown of your head to your feet, *dristi: padhayoragrai*.

Jump Back into full Vinyasa or Half Vinyasa

The full vinyasa between each completed posture and the half vinyasa between each side of the posture are essential for maintaining the internal heat of the body, which allows the muscles and joints to be deeply stretched and opened safely. The jump back cultivates co-ordination between the body and mind, and develops upper body strength.

Jump Back

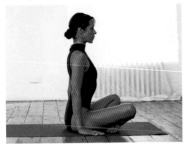

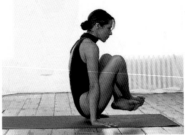

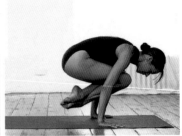

From **Dandasana** (staff posture), cross your ankles and *exhale*, placing your palms down on the floor by the sides of your hips. Deepen uddiyana bandha to prepare for the next step, and shift your shoulders forwards over your wrists.

⟶ *Inhale* and press your hands strongly into the floor. Use the power and strength of uddiyana bandha to curl the front of your torso up slightly. Press through your arms into your palms and raise your buttocks and feet off the floor into **Lolasana** (tremulous posture).

⟶ Continue to *inhale* and without touching the floor, swing your feet back and your head and chest forwards into advanced **Lolasana** (tremulous posture) moving your shoulders forwards of your wrists right over your fingertips.

Full Vinyasa

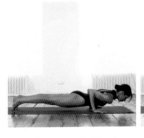

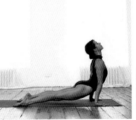

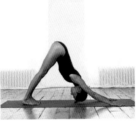

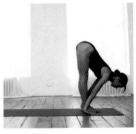

Exhale, jump your feet back into **Chaturanga Dandasana**.

⟶ *Inhale* to stretch into **Urdhva Mukha Svanasana**.

⟶ *Exhale* and move into **Adho Mukha Svanasana**.

⟶ *Inhale*, jump your feet into **Urdhva Uttanasana**.

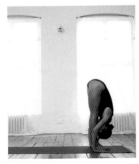

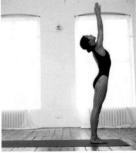

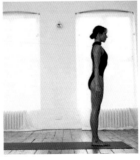

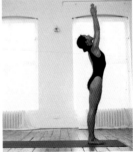

⟶ *Exhale* and fold into **Uttanasana**.

⟶ *Inhale* stretching into **Urdhva Tadasana**.

⟶ *Exhale*, lowering your arms into **Tadasana**.

⟶ *Inhale*, stretch up into **Urdhva Tadasana**.

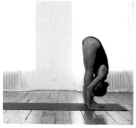

→ *Exhale* and fold forwards into **Uttanasana**

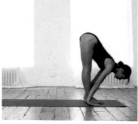

→ *Inhale* and lift your chest into **Urdhva Uttanasana**.

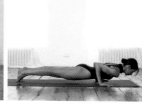

→ *Exhale* and jump into **Chaturanga Dandasana**.

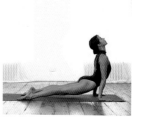

→ *Inhale* and stretch into **Urdhva Mukha Svanasana**.

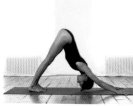

→ *Exhale* and move into **Adho Mukha Svanasana**.

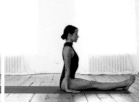

→ *Inhale* and jump through into **Dandasana**

Benefits of the vinyasa
The sequence of the full vinyasa is practised after having completed a seated posture on both sides. The half vinyasa is practised in between sides of each posture. As well as sustaining the heat of the muscles and the flow of the body, vinyasas neutralize and align the body, preparing it for the next posture. You may wish to refer back to Surya Namaskara for extra details of the transition through the postures of vinyasa.

Jump back into Half Vinyasa

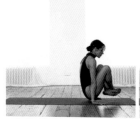

Inhale, press down through your arms and raise your seat off the floor.

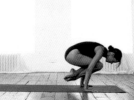

→ Continuing to *inhale*, move into **Lolasana** (see step 3 of jump back).

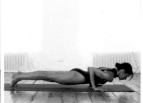

→ *Exhale* and jump your feet back into **Chaturanga Dandasana**.

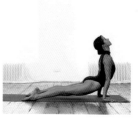

→ *Inhale* and stretch into **Urdhva Mukha Svanasana**.

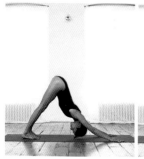

→ *Exhale* and move into **Adho Mukha Svanasana**.

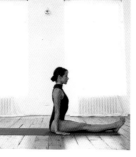

→ *Inhale* and jump through into **Dandasana**.

Easing into the vinyasa
The swing into Lolasana is a very challenging movement, so initially begin to practise this by crossing your ankles and placing your hands on the ground in front of your shins. From here, softly roll forwards over your feet to take your weight into your hands, and then jump or step back into Chaturanga

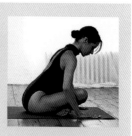

Dandasana. Once you have gained confidence, try to lift your buttocks off the floor.

Pūrvottānāsana | STRETCH OF THE EAST POSTURE

purva = east (which represents the front in yoga)
uttana = extended or intense stretch

In this complete counter-posture to Paschimottanasana the front of the body is lengthened and stretched open, lifting the heart above the level of the spine. This increases the blood flow to the brain, refreshing and revitalizing body and mind.

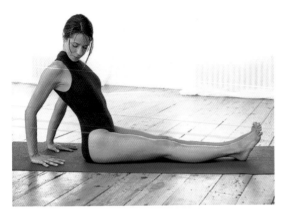

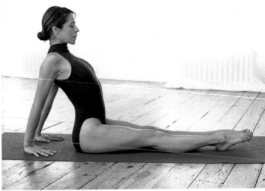

1 From Dandasana, *exhale* and step your hands back behind your hips, planting your palms into the floor with your fingers pointing inwards towards your buttocks.

2 Draw the back of your waist up and in, while strongly lifting your chest up to your chin and rolling your shoulders back. Stretch your legs long, extending out to your toes.

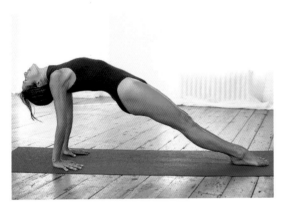

3 *Inhale* and press your hands deeper into the floor, propelling your hips upwards as you extend your toes and the balls of your feet downwards. Raise your heart higher and release your neck, allowing your head to drop softly back. Stretch your legs long and together, keeping them active and rooting your big-toe joints down. *Take five to ten breaths*, expanding your chest and focusing towards your nose tip, <u>dristi</u>: **nasagrai**. *Exhale*, lower your buttocks to the floor and lift your head up, returning to Dandasana.

• *Inhale*, press your hands into the floor, tuck your knees up, crossing your ankles, and lift your hips off the floor to swing your feet back into a **full vinyasa**. Flow through the vinyasa and then softly **jump through** and return to Dandasana.

Deepening the pose
Make sure your hands are placed shoulder-width apart and spread your fingers open. Work the rotation in your shoulders and broaden across your chest. Lift your tailbone in and up towards your pubic bone and feel your spine pressing up into the front of your torso.

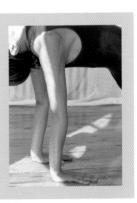

Easing into the pose
If at first you can't get a good lift bend your knees and step your feet apart, both flat on the floor. From here, raise your pelvis and create a parallel line to the floor with your torso.

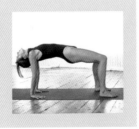

Ardha Baddha Padma Paschimottānāsana | HALF BOUND LOTUS INTENSE STRETCH OF THE WEST POSTURE

ardha = half
baddha = bound or caught
padma = lotus paschima = west
uttana = extended or intense stretch

The full folding of one leg at a time opens the knee joints, preparing them for the full lotus (Padmasana), which forms part of the seated sequence. This posture massages the abdominal organs, improving both digestion and elimination.

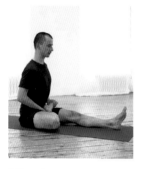
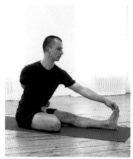

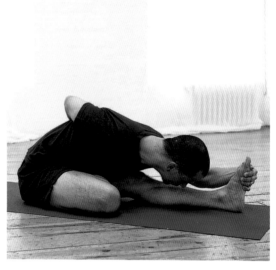

1 From landing in Dandasana from your full vinyasa, continue to *inhale*, folding your right knee and using your hands to draw your right foot up and on to your left upper thigh. Place the little-toe edge of your foot into the crease of your left hip socket. Align your heel just above your pubic bone and move your right knee forwards and in, to create a 45-degree angle with your left leg. Keep your left leg actively lengthening out through its heel, as your right leg is now in half lotus (Ardha Padma).

2 *Towards the end of your inhalation*, stretch your right arm behind your back and catch hold of your right big toe with the first two fingers of your right hand. Extend your left hand to hold your left foot and lengthen your spine.

3 *Exhale slowly* and lengthen your back forwards out from your hips, moving your chest towards your left knee and your chin towards your left shin. Softly bend your left elbow wide to the side, drawing your abdomen long over your right heel, and *breathe five to ten long, even breaths* while sending energy and focus out to your extended foot, <u>dristi</u>: **padhayoragrai**. *Inhale*, lift your chest up, *exhale* and release the bind of your hands from your feet and stretch your right leg forwards into Dandasana.

• *Inhale*, press your hands into the floor, tuck your knees up, crossing your ankles, and lift your hips off the floor to move into a **half vinyasa**. Return to Dandasana. Repeat this posture, this time folding your left leg into half lotus. After *five to ten breaths*, take a **full vinyasa** and **jump through** to Dandasana.

Easing into the pose

If strain is felt in your knees, do not force the posture. Instead, either remain upright and work on relaxing your hips to allow the knee to release and drop closer to the floor, or take your foot to the ground and softly extend your body forwards from here. Use a strap in either of these positions if you are not yet able to reach hold of your foot.

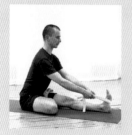
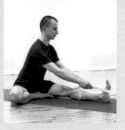

Deepening the pose

Soften the skin over your bent knee to allow the joint to fully bend. Now gently press your knee downwards to further the rotation of your leg and the opening in your hip. Move your lower abdomen forwards and down on to the lotus heel (of your bent leg) to stimulate the abdominal organs.

Triaṅg Mukhaikapāda Paschimottānāsana | THREE LIMBS FACE ONE LEG INTENSE STRETCH OF THE WEST POSTURE

tri = three
anga = limb
mukha = face
eka = one

pada = foot/leg
paschima = west
uttana = intense
stretch

The three "limbs" referred to are the feet (stretching forwards and backwards), the knees (which are opened) and the buttocks (which are drawn wide as the back extends forwards). This posture also provides a counter-stretch to the previous half lotus.

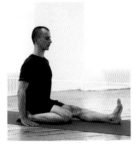
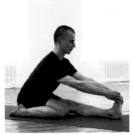

1 From landing in Dandasana from your full vinyasa, continue to *inhale* and bend your right knee, taking your right foot back. Place your heel against your right hip, with the front of your right foot, ankle and shinbone pressing on the floor. Join your knees together and root down evenly into both sitting bones, pressing both buttocks firmly down.

2 At the *end of your inhalation*, open your chest wide, extend your back long and tilt your pelvis forwards, stretching your arms out and catching hold of your left foot with both your hands.

Benefits of the pose
Triang Mukhaikapada Paschimottanasana is particularly helpful for releasing tightness in the back of the pelvis. It also opens the sacrum area to stimulate and improve circulation throughout the nerves (especially the sciatic nerve) of the spine and the muscles of the back.

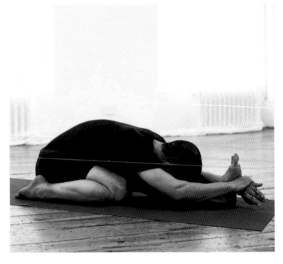

3 *Exhale* and fold deeper from your hips, sending your pubic bone back and down and lengthening your torso out and over your left leg. Stretch along your spine and draw the top of your head towards your toes, bending your elbows outwards. Sink your right buttock and hip downwards to maintain an even base for this posture. *Take five to ten breaths* and focus on sending energy out to your extended foot, **dristi: padhayoragrai**. *Inhale*, maintaining the hold of your foot, and draw your chest up, rolling your shoulders back. *Exhale*, release your hands from your foot and bring your body upright, extending your right leg forwards into Dandasana.

• *Inhale*, press your hands into the floor, tuck your knees up, crossing your ankles, and lift your hips off the floor to swing your feet back. Move smoothly through a **half vinyasa** and then **jump through**, landing gently into Dandasana. Repeat this posture, this time bending your left leg. After *five to ten breaths*, take a **full vinyasa** and **jump through** to land softly into Dandasana.

Easing into the pose
Always be aware of pain in the knees, as this may be an indication of working too deeply too quickly. If this is the case, place a firm cushion, folded blanket or yoga block under the buttock of your straight leg. This will not only help to protect the knee but will also assist in rooting both buttocks squarely. Again, with this pose use a strap to

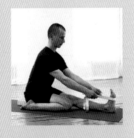

catch your foot if you tend to bend your leg or hunch your back in order to hold it with your hands.

Deepening the pose
To deepen the openness across your sacrum, roll your inner thighs together and downwards; this will also develop the full range of leg rotation. As you do this, be sure to engage uddiyana bandha to support your lower spine.

Jānu Śīrṣāsana A | KNEE HEAD POSTURE A

janu = knee
sirsa = head

This posture provides the foundation of the following two variations and continues to open the pelvis and develop the suppleness and freedom of the hips and knees. It balances and tones the liver and spleen, so improving the digestive system.

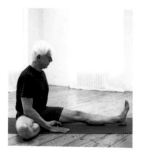
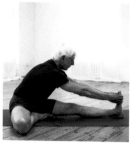

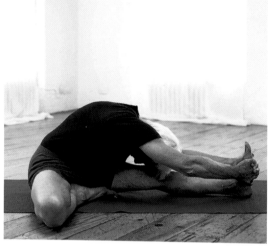

1 From landing in Dandasana out of your full vinyasa, continue to *inhale* and bend your right knee back in line with, or slightly behind, your right shoulder (at 90–95 degrees to your left leg). Place your right heel so that it touches its own inner upper thigh, as this will ensure a full opening in your right hip. Square your body to face your left leg, with your navel in line with your left knee.

2 At the *end of your inhalation*, extend your back forwards from your pelvis and reach your hands out to catch hold of your left foot, keeping your collarbones open and your shoulders relaxed.

3 *Exhale* and deepen the fold at the level of your hips, extending your torso out over your left leg. Gently press your right knee and outer thigh down on to the floor, and stretch your left heel away to lengthen through your left leg. Draw your shoulders away from your hands, and softly bend your elbows wide, pressing your chest forwards to your left knee. *Take five to ten even breaths* and direct focus and energy out to your extended foot, <u>dristi: **padhayoragrai**</u>. *Inhale*, maintaining hold of your foot, straighten your arms and draw your chest up, drawing your shoulders back and down. *Exhale*, release the hold of your foot and bring your torso upright, extending your right leg forwards into Dandasana.

• *Inhale*, press your hands into the floor, tuck your knees up, crossing your ankles, and lift your hips off the floor. Move smoothly through a **half vinyasa** and **jump through**, landing gently into Dandasana. Repeat this posture, this time bending your left leg. After *five to ten breaths*, take a **full vinyasa** and **jump through** into Dandasana.

Easing into the pose
It is better to work initially with a strap to link your hands to your foot if you feel that you are not yet able to hold your toes with a straight back and leg. Using a strap will help to prevent you from straining your shoulders and rounding your back.

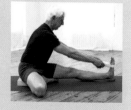

Concentrate on lengthening your spine at all times within this pose.

Deepening the pose
Focus on both sides of your torso being level so that your back expands open and receives an even stretch. This will help to balance the kidneys and the muscle flexibility of the back. With each exhalation, yield the open expanse of your back to gravity.

Jānu Śīrṣāsana B | KNEE HEAD POSTURE B

janu = knee
sirsa = head

In this variation of Janu Sirsasana, the heel is pressed underneath the perineum, helping to maintain the activity of mula bandha. Sitting on the foot also helps to tilt the pelvis forwards, thus enabling a deeper forwards stretch through the body.

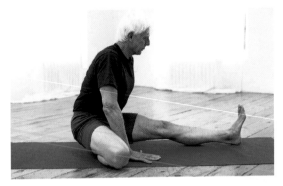

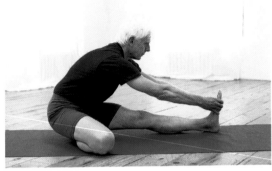

1 From Dandasana, continue to *inhale* as you bend your right knee back, moving your right foot towards the pubis. Press down on your hands to raise your hips, then shift your pelvis forwards, placing your perineum on top of your right heel. Direct the toes of your right foot forwards to your left heel and place your right knee at an 80-degree angle to your left leg.

2 At the *end of your inhalation*, widen your collarbones and extend your back forwards, pivoting from your pelvis and holding your left foot with both hands.

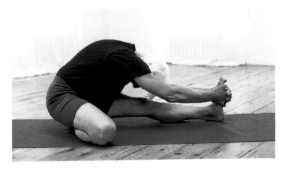

3 *Exhale* and softly fold from your hips to stretch your torso forwards over your left leg, bending your elbows wide and lengthening through the back of your neck. Keep centring the front of your body directly over your left leg. Extend your left heel away and draw your left thigh muscle upwards and in towards your hip. Focus on sending energy out to your extended foot, <u>dristi</u>: **padhayoragrai**, and *take five full breaths*. *Inhale* and draw your chest up, keeping your hands held around your foot, and straighten your arms. *Exhale* and bring your torso upright, extending your right leg into Dandasana.

• *Inhale*, press your hands into the floor, tuck your knees up, crossing your ankles, and lift your hips off the floor. Flow through a **half vinyasa** and then softly **jump through** into Dandasana. Repeat this posture, this time bending your left leg. After *five to ten breaths*, take a **full vinyasa** and **jump through** to land softly into Dandasana.

Benefits of the pose
In addition to the overall positive effects of the Janu Sirsasana variations for both men and women alike, this posture is of particular benefit to men. The placement of the heel against the perineum and the stretch through the pelvis helps to regulate the prostate gland, protecting against its enlargement. Those who have this condition are advised to stay longer in this asana.

Easing into the pose
Use a strap if you have difficulty in reaching your extended foot. If the underside of your foot feels uncomfortable, folding your mat under it may help to cushion the bones.

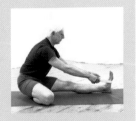

Deepening the pose
Feel the connection of your perineum with your heel at all times throughout this asana. Anchor into this point and release your torso forwards and out, away from this base of mula bandha.

Jānu Śīrṣāsana C | KNEE HEAD POSTURE C

janu = knee
sirsa = head

In this final and deepest posture of the Janu Sirsasana variations, the entire leg, and its potential mobility and power, is fully stimulated from the hip to the toes, improving circulation and energy flow from the pelvis through the hips down into the legs.

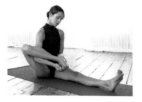
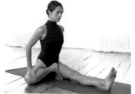

1 From Dandasana, continue to *inhale* as you bend your right leg, taking your right elbow under your right knee and holding your right toes. With your left hand, press your right heel forwards, then place your right toes and ball of the foot by your left inner thigh at a 45-degree angle. Keep your right heel lifting up and move the arch of your right foot to your left inner thigh.

2 With your foot in place, release your hands from your right foot and gently rotate your right knee forwards and down to the floor.

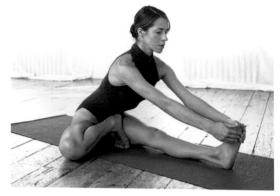

3 At the *end of your inhalation*, lengthen your back forwards, folding from your pelvis, and stretch your abdominal wall long to create length from your pubis to your navel. Raise your abdomen and navel up and over your right heel, extending your hands to hold your left foot.

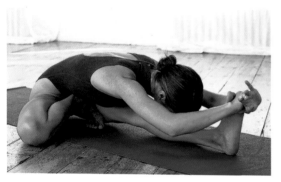

4 *Exhale* and extend your torso out along your left leg, bending your elbows out. Maintain length throughout your spine and back of your neck as you direct the top of your head towards your left ankle. Be active in your left leg and softly open the back of your left thigh, knee and calf down into the floor. *Take five to ten deep breaths*, fully engaging uddiyana bandha, and focus on sending energy out to your extended foot, <u>dristi</u>: padhayoragrai, while rooting into both sitting bones. *Inhale* and draw your chest up, rolling your shoulders back and straightening your arms while still holding your foot. *Exhale* and bring your back upright, releasing your right leg into Dandasana.

• *Inhale*, press your hands into the floor, tuck your knees up, cross your ankles and lift your hips off the floor. Move smoothly through a **half vinyasa** and then softly **jump through** into Dandasana. Repeat this posture, this time with your left leg bending in. After *five to ten breaths*, take a **full vinyasa** and **jump through** to land softly into Dandasana.

Benefits of the pose
This particular placement of the foot opens the toe joints, stretches the muscles of the soles and creates suppleness in the ankle joints. As the bent knee descends, an opening of the hip and knee is created and the Achilles tendon and calf muscle are lengthened.

Easing into the pose
This is a strong posture and so must be approached with care, patience and intelligence. The rotation of the leg and knee originates within your hip socket, so do not strain or force your knee down. With careful practice the hips will gradually release, allowing your knee to descend and your torso to lean over your straight leg. Be content to work just at stage 1 or 2 until your body is ready to go further.

Deepening the pose
As your bent knee descends, it is easy for your base to become unbalanced, which will distort the alignment and posture of your body. Focus on cultivating an even awareness of gravity rooting you into both sitting bones.

Marīchyāsana A | POSTURE A DEDICATED TO THE GREAT SAGE MARICHI

Marichi = the son of Brahma (the creator) and grandfather of Surya (the sun god)

In this forward extension of the torso, the hands are bound behind the back. This means that the movement of the abdomen inwards to deepen uddiyana bandha and the yielding to gravity are both essential to extend the torso forwards and down.

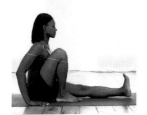
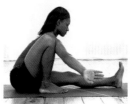
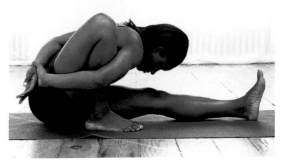

1 From Dandasana, continue to *inhale* slowly, and bend your right knee up towards your right shoulder. Place your right heel firmly on the ground in line with your right sitting bone, with your right toes pointing directly forwards.

2 Continue to *inhale*, and reach your right arm and hand out, with the palm facing away from your body. Move your right outer shoulder to the inside of your right knee, and place your left hand on the floor by your left hip.

3 Towards the *end of your inhalation*, sweep your right arm around to the right side, opening your right armpit against the front of your right shinbone. Take your hands back to clasp behind your back. Lengthen your spine and open your chest while squaring your shoulders forwards.

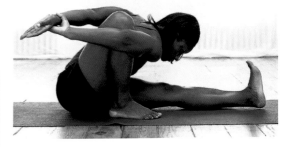

Easing into the pose
When you first learn this posture you may not be able to bind your hands, so instead use a strap to link your hands behind your back. As you practise, gradually walk your fingers closer together along the strap until they touch.

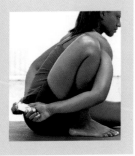

Deepening the pose
Bind your hands securely, as this will create a loop of energy through your arms and help to seal you into the posture. As the binding of your fingers becomes easier and your body more supple, on the first side of this asana use your right hand to hold your left wrist, and on the second side use your left hand to hold your right wrist. Once this is possible, stretch your arms, raising your hands up and away from your back.

4 *Exhale* and extend your torso out and over your left leg, folding deep within your hips. Stretch your left heel away and press your right inner thigh against the side of your right ribcage. Point your right knee directly up. Breathe length into your back and draw your chest open towards your left knee, extending your arms out behind you. *Take five to ten breaths*, deeply engaging uddiyana bandha and focusing energy out to your extended foot, **dristi: padhayoragrai**. *Inhale*, raise your chest and open your shoulders wide. *Exhale* and release the bind of your hands, bringing your body upright and stretching your right leg forwards into Dandasana.

• *Inhale*, press your hands into the floor, tuck your knees up, cross your ankles and lift your hips off the floor. Move smoothly through a **half vinyasa** and then softly **jump through** into Dandasana. Repeat this posture, this time folding your left knee in. After *five to ten breaths*, take a **full vinyasa** and **jump through** to land softly into Dandasana.

Marichi = the son of Brahma (the creator) and grandfather of Surya (the sun god)

This asana intensifies the benefits of Marichyasana A, as the heel of the lotus leg applies pressure to the abdomen, helping to stimulate, massage and tone the internal organs. The pose also releases tension from the shoulders.

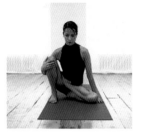

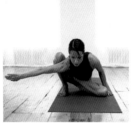

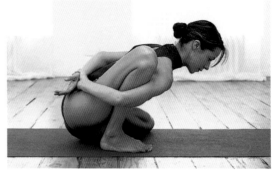

1 From landing in Dandasana from your full vinyasa, continue to *inhale*, bending your left leg, and use your hands to draw your left foot up and on to your right upper thigh into half lotus. Move the little-toe edge of your left foot into the crease of your right hip socket, then release your left hand on to the floor. Sit on your left buttock, drawing your left knee and thigh down. Bend your right knee up towards your right shoulder and place your right heel on the ground in line with your right sitting bone. Direct your right toes to point forwards.

2 Continue to *inhale* and extend your torso forwards over your left foot, moving your right shoulder to the inside of your right knee and beyond. Stretch your right arm out to the side to place your right armpit on the front of your right shin.

3 Towards the *end of your inhalation*, fold your right arm around your right leg, taking both hands backwards to catch hold together behind your back. Extend out through your spine, lifting your chest and squaring your shoulders.

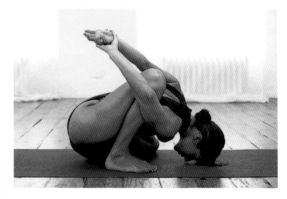

Easing into the pose
Progress through this posture slowly, being extremely careful of your knees. If you experience any pain, ease off and release the lotus foot on to the floor and practise the posture here.

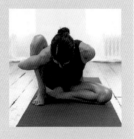

Deepening the pose
As you progress in this posture, concentrate on fully engaging uddiyana, which will help you to extend your torso further forwards and your head lower. As this begins to happen, you will be able to bind at your wrists and raise your hands as in Marichyasana A.

4 *Exhale* and stretch your torso forwards and over your left heel, drawing your head towards the floor and directing your chin in between and beyond your knee and foot. Press your right inner thigh into the right side of your ribcage, directing the kneecap upwards. *Take five to ten full, even breaths*, releasing the back of your neck long and looking towards your nose tip, <u>dristi: nasagrai</u>. *Inhale*, raise your chest and open your shoulders wide. *Exhale* and release the bind of your hands, bringing your body upright and stretching your legs forwards into Dandasana (staff posture).

• *Inhale*, press your hands into the floor, tuck your knees up, cross your ankles and lift your hips off the floor to swing your feet back. Flow through the **half vinyasa** and then **jump through** into Dandasana. Repeat this posture, this time folding your right knee into half lotus. After *five to ten breaths*, take a **full vinyasa** and **jump through** to land softly into Dandasana.

Marīchyāsana C | POSTURE C DEDICATED TO THE GREAT SAGE MARICHI

Marichi = the son of Brahma
(the creator) and grandfather
of Surya (the sun god)

The two previous asanas have increased the blood flow to flush through the internal organs, and now these two twists of Marichyasana C and D squeeze out any toxins from the abdomen, which can create imbalances and sluggishness of digestion.

SEATED ASANAS

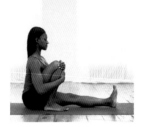

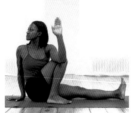

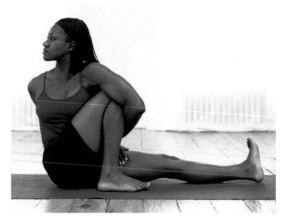

1 From landing in Dandasana from your full vinyasa, continue to *inhale*, and bend your right knee up towards your right shoulder. Place the heel firmly on the ground in line with your right sitting bone, with your right toes pointing directly forwards, as in Marichyasana A. Lengthen your back and softly press your torso forwards to your right thigh.

2 Continue to *inhale*, stretching your back taller, and take your right hand on to the floor behind your pelvis. Open your right shoulder back and draw your right knee inwards to the centre of your chest. Turn your chest to your right leg, then hook your left elbow and armpit over your right knee and move the left side of your ribs into your right inner thigh. Roll the right side of your ribs back.

3 Continue to *inhale* and extend your left hand out so your palm turns down and your elbow rolls up. Now wrap your bent left arm around your right bent leg. Take your right hand off the floor to catch hold of your left hand. Draw your right shoulder back, turning your head to bring your chin over your right shoulder. *Take five to ten breaths*, looking over your right shoulder, <u>**dristi: parsva**</u>. With each *inhalation*, breathe length into your spine and openness into your chest. With each exhalation, draw your right shoulder back and down, turning your collarbone and side ribs further around to the right. *Exhale*, release the clasp of your hands and return your body to face forwards, stretching your legs out into Dandasana.

• *Inhale*, press your hands into the floor, tuck your knees up, cross your ankles and lift your hips off the floor to swing your feet back. Flow through a **half vinyasa** and then **jump through** to land gently into Dandasana. Repeat this posture, this time bending your left leg up. After *five to ten breaths*, take a **full vinyasa** and **jump through** to land softly into Dandasana.

Benefits of the pose
Twists are a wonderful tonic for the spine, bringing about spinal health, balance and mobility, as well as helping to alleviate back stiffness and pain.

Easing into the pose
Binding in this posture takes time, as it requires and develops not just full mobility and suppleness but also a good deal of strength throughout the back muscles. Be prepared, therefore, to work this posture only to stage 2 until the body develops sufficient flexibility and control. If you suffer from particular tightness in the back, you may find sitting

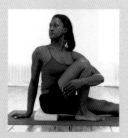

on a firm cushion or yoga block beneficial to help prevent your back from collapsing and dropping backwards.

Deepening the pose
As the rotation through your spine develops, you will be able to bind at your wrists and so rotate further. Note that the left hand holds the right wrist and the right fingers stretch to the left inner thigh (and vice versa on the second side).

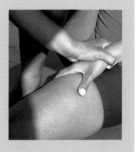

Marīchyāsana D | POSTURE D DEDICATED TO THE GREAT SAGE MARICHI

Marichi = the son of the Brahma (the creator) and grandfather of Surya (the sun god)

This final twist develops the flexibility and mobility of the spine and back muscles that were introduced in Marichyasana C. One side of the back and abdomen is squeezed, while the other side is stretched, releasing tension and stress from the spinal nerves.

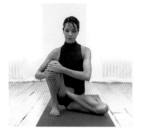 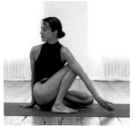

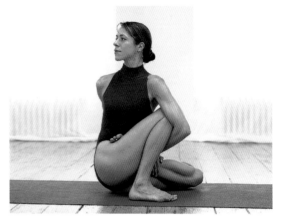

1 From landing in Dandasana from your full vinyasa, continue to *inhale*, drawing your left leg and foot up into half lotus. Sit on to your left buttock and draw your left knee and thigh down. Bend your right knee up and place your right heel on the ground in line with your right sitting bone, as in Marichyasana B. Strongly draw your back tall and your chest up.

2 Continue to *inhale*, lengthening your spine and drawing your right knee across to the centre of your chest, then move your chest to your right knee. Now lean forwards and rotate through your back to hook your left upper arm firmly over your right knee and move your left armpit over on to your right outer knee. Press the left side of your ribs into your right inner thigh, rolling the right side of your torso back. Place your right hand on the floor behind your pelvis, rolling your right shoulder open and extending your left hand forwards.

3 Towards the end of your *inhalation*, twist fully through your spine, and, while pressing your left ribs forwards into your right leg, wrap your left arm around your right leg and then reach your left hand to the left side of your waist. Draw your right shoulder open and stretch your right hand back to grasp your left hand. As you *exhale*, open your right shoulder, turning your head to look over your right shoulder, **dristi: parsva**. *Take five to ten breaths*. Focus on lifting through the entire length of your spine, drawing your chest skywards and sliding your shoulder blades down your back. *Exhale*, release the bind of your hands, returning your body to face forwards, and stretch your legs into Dandasana.

• *Inhale*, press your hands into the floor, tuck your knees up, cross your ankles and lift your hips off the floor to swing your feet back. Flow through the **half vinyasa** and then **jump through** to land gently into Dandasana. Repeat the posture, this time bending your left leg up. After *five to ten breaths*, take a **full vinyasa** and **jump through** to land softly into Dandasana.

Easing into the pose
If initially you are unable to clasp your hands, build up to the binding by hugging into your leg. If your knees are not strong enough for deep lotus work, you can moderate the posture by placing your left foot on the floor close to your right buttock, as in Marichyasana B, and

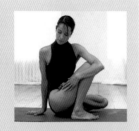

practise twisting your spine from this moderated positioning of your legs.

Deepening the pose
To deepen the rotation of your spine, focus (while on the first side) on moving your left ribcage forwards into your right thigh to close any gap between the two, and draw your right ribcage backwards. This will also enable you to bind at the wrist, taking your fingers on to the shin. In turn, this will

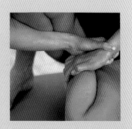

increase the heel pressure against your abdomen, so intensifying the benefits.

Nāvāsana and Lolāsana | BOAT POSTURE AND TREMULOUS POSTURE

nava = boat
lola = dangling or swaying like a pendulum

Individually, these postures cultivate bandha awareness and develop bandha control. When practised together, they develop abdominal and leg tone, back strength, and power in the arms, wrists and shoulders.

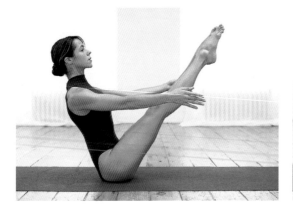

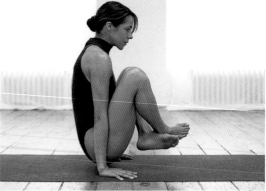

1 From landing in Dandasana from your full vinyasa, continue to *inhale*, reclining your chest back and upwards at the same time as lifting your legs up, with your inner thighs, ankles and big-toe joints pressing together. Stretch your legs and ankles long, raise your arms horizontally and reach your hands forwards beyond your knees. Float your feet upwards as high as your head, and balance on your buttocks, not allowing your back to collapse down on to the floor. *Take five breaths* in Navasana, looking towards your toes, **dristi: padhayoragrai**.

2 *Exhale* and move into Lolasana by placing your palms down on the floor by the sides of your hips and deepening uddiyana bandha to curl and contract the front of your torso. Shift your shoulders forwards over your wrists. *Inhale* and press your hands strongly into the floor, then, using the power and strength of uddiyana bandha and the pressure down through your arms into your palms, raise your buttocks and feet off the floor, tucking your legs in tightly. This is Lolasana. *Exhale softly*, lower your buttocks back down on to the floor and stretch in to Navasana, and *take five breaths*. *Exhale*, place your palms down on the floor by the sides of your hips and lift up into Lolasana. Repeat three more times so that you practise Navasana and Lolasana five times in all.

• From your fifth Lolasana jump your feet back into Chaturanga Dandasana and move through a **full vinyasa**. From the Adho Mukha Svanasana of the vinyasa, instead of jumping through to land into Dandasana, jump and gently land on your feet in front of your hands, as shown on the next page.

Easing into the pose
These two poses are challenging. Pace yourself by breathing slowly and deeply. If your lower back feels strained in Navasana, bend your knees, lowering your feet so that your shins are parallel to the floor.

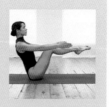

Deepening the pose
As you become proficient in Lolasana, try swinging your feet back, raising your hips over your shoulders and hands, and then stretching your legs up into a full handstand balance as you inhale. To return to Navasana, slowly exhale, tuck your legs in and, with bandha control, gently swing your pelvis back down to Lolasana, then place your buttocks down into Navasana. Practise this five times. This deeper pose combats fatigue and refreshes the nervous system.

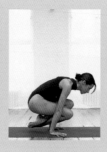

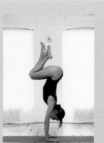

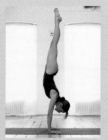

Bhujapīdāsana | ARM PRESSURE POSTURE

bhuja = arm or shoulder
pida = pressure

This pose creates strength in the hands and wrists, leanness in the muscles of the arms and increased flexibility in the shoulder joints. When the legs are drawn up towards the torso, this helps to balance the pancreas and the secretion of insulin.

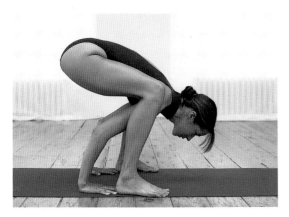

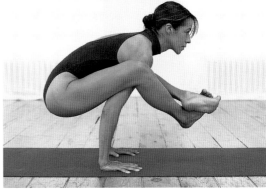

1 From the Adho Mukha Svanasana of your full vinyasa, *inhale* and jump your feet forwards of your hands, with your legs to the outside of your arms and your knees by your shoulders. Continue to *inhale* and deepen the bend of your knees, lowering the back of your thighs towards your inner upper arms. Spread your palms and fingers open, and extend your middle fingers to your heels.

2 Towards the *end of your inhalation*, place the back of your thighs on to your upper arms. Shift your weight back on to your hands, without dropping your buttocks down, and lift your feet from the floor, crossing your ankles. Lift your face and softly gaze towards your nose tip, **dristi: nasagrai**.

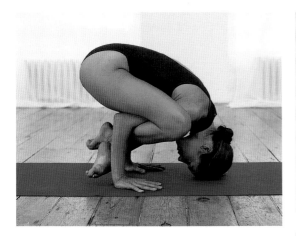

Easing into the pose
In order to get your shoulders far enough back, bend your knees deeply, then step your hands on to the back of your ankles and move your shoulders towards the back of your knees. Work gently and with patience, gradually building confidence to take your full weight on your hands. If at first you cannot

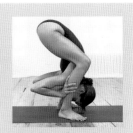

lift both feet at once, practise lifting one foot at a time, then lift both and work to cross your ankles.

3 *Exhale*, tip your head and shoulders forwards and down, bringing your forehead towards the floor, and, at the same time, strongly work uddiyana to send your feet and buttocks back and upwards. This is like a seesaw action into a balance point. *Take five to ten breaths*, looking to your nose tip, **dristi: nasagrai**. From here, *inhale*, raise your face and chest and return to step 2. Then uncross your ankles, and either place your feet on the floor and **jump back** into Chaturanga Dandasana to enter into a **full vinyasa** or stretch your legs into Tittibhasana and then Bakasana, as overleaf, to enter into a **full vinyasa**.

Deepening the pose
Instead of landing on your feet, jump your legs directly into Tittibhasana, then bend your knees, cross your ankles and lower your head into Bhujapidasana. As you gain strength, extend your chin to the floor.

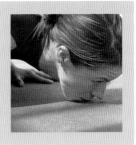

Ṭiṭṭibhāsana and Bakāsana | FIREFLY POSTURE AND CRANE POSTURE

tittibha = firefly
baka = crane bird

These asanas together create a seamless transition from Bhujapidasana into a full vinyasa. Tittibhasana stretches the spinal cord and back while extending length and power into the legs. Bakasana helps to develop the strength required for a handstand.

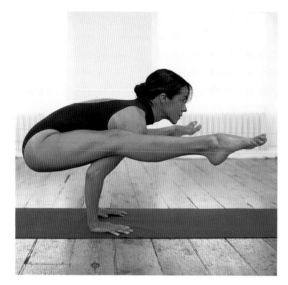

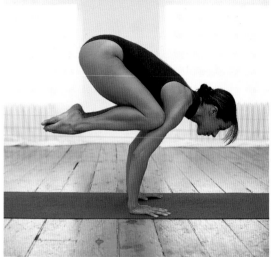

1 From Bhujapidasana, *inhale*, raise your face and chest, uncrossing your ankles and stretching your legs forwards. Extend out through the balls of your feet into Tittibhasana. Maintain the pressure of your inner thighs against your upper arms and press your palms strongly down into the ground. Deeply engage uddiyana bandha. Draw strength up through your arms, lift your buttocks, chest and face so that you hover parallel to the floor. Look towards your nosetip, **dristi: nasagrai**.

2 Begin to *exhale*, and engage uddiyana bandha even deeper. Raise your hips, keeping your chest open and your head forwards as you fold at your knees, and take your shins, ankles and feet back into Bakasana. Bring your big toes together and lift your heels towards your buttocks. *Inhale*, feeling the support of your arms and uddiyana and mula bandha. Roll your shoulders back and lengthen the back of your neck. Look towards your nose tip, **dristi: nasagrai**.

• *Exhale* and shoot your feet backwards, bending your elbows as your feet land into Chaturanga Dandasana. From here flow into a **full vinyasa**. Do not jump through into Dandasana, but as in the vinyasa after Navasana and Lolasana jump your feet onto the floor by your hands (page 87).

Benefits of the pose
The linking together of these two asanas enhances co-ordination, grace and dynamic energy. They harness the energy of the bandhas and tone the abdominal muscles, internal organs and inner thighs to create a sense of poise and balance.

Easing into the pose
This transition may take some practice to accomplish and complete, so as always be patient. At first you may wish to focus on attaining Tittibhasana before attempting Bakasana. Once you feel strong and confident in the first posture, then work towards Bakasana. Try bending one leg back at a time, gradually building the strength to take both feet back together in a smooth motion.

Deepening the pose
As you become more adept in this sweeping, bird-like transition, before springing back into Chaturanga Dandasana raise your knees off your arms with an inhalation and then shoot your feet back to continue into the full vinyasa with your next exhalation. As you practise this transition physical lightness and agility is cultivated and the entire body is toned and strengthened.

Kurmasana | TORTOISE POSTURE

Kurma = tortoise incarnation of Visnu, preserver of the universe, second deity of the Hindu trinity

This posture intensely lengthens the back muscles and releases tightness in the lumbar region and sacrum, allowing energy to flow freely through the spine. If uddiyana is fully engaged, both respiratory and digestive systems are improved.

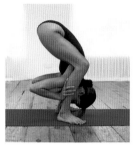 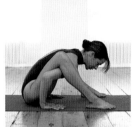

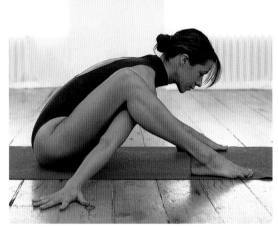

1 From the Adho Mukha Svanasana of your full vinyasa, *inhale* and jump your feet on to the floor forwards of your hands, with your legs to the outside of your arms and your knees by your shoulders, as you did to enter into Bhujapidasana. Take your hands to the backs of your ankles and move your shoulders to the backs of your knees.

2 Continue to *inhale* and bend your knees deeply and soften in your hips. Place your hands on the floor and lower your buttocks on to the floor. Deepen your engagement of uddiyana bandha to control the lowering of your hips into a gentle descent.

3 Stretch your arms out underneath your knees, extending through your fingertips out to the sides, and gently draw the backs of your knees over to the very tops of your arms.

4 As you *complete your inhalation*, deepen the fold in the front of your hips, stretch your legs long while firmly pressing your heels forwards. This straightening of your legs will press down on the backs of your upper arms and shoulders which will help descend your torso closer to the floor. Open your chest wide and forwards along the floor and move your pubic bone back and down as you reach out through your arms. Draw your abdomen wall long, and lengthen through the front of your spine and throat to lay your ribs and chin on the floor. Look towards your third eye, <u>dristi</u>: **bru madhya**, and *take five to ten full, deep breaths* in this asana, before moving into the profound posture of Supta Kurmasana.

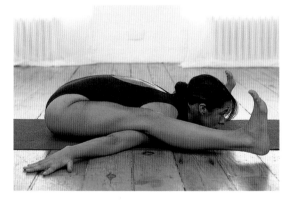

Easing into the pose
Work step by step to press your heels away gradually in order to straighten your legs. If this causes a sensation of overpulling in your back, keep your knees bent and softly release your torso forwards as in step 3. Then, each time you practise this pose, gently move your feet further forwards until sufficient suppleness is developed within your hips and leg muscles to allow you to extend your legs forwards into the complete posture.

Deepening the pose
Each time you exhale in this asana, feel the fold at the front of your hips receding further backwards and in towards your buttock bones. Send energy out along the backs of your legs through into your heels, while drawing your thigh muscles up and in towards your front hips. This will help to create full length and strength in your leg muscles so that your legs straighten and your heels rise off the ground as the front of your torso opens into the ground.

Supta Kūrmāsana | SLEEPING TORTOISE POSTURE

supta = sleeping
Kurma = tortoise incarnation of
Visnu, preserver of the universe,
second deity of the Hindu trinity

This asana is physically completed by bowing the head low, and mentally completed by the drawing in of the mind, inducing introspection, stillness, inner calm and a quiet surrender to universal flow.

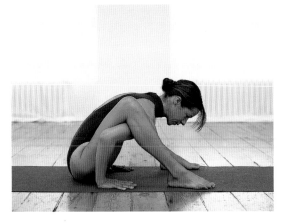

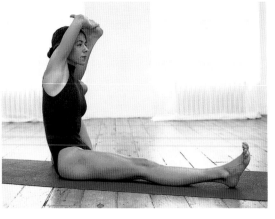

1 From Kurmasana, *inhale* and raise your head from the floor, bending your knees to release your arms and pressing your palms down under your shoulders to draw your torso up.

2 *Exhale* and bringing your body upright, catch hold of your left foot with your right hand, bending your left knee up and back behind your left shoulder. *Inhale*, opening your chest. Press your left shoulder back to help move your left thigh and knee back.

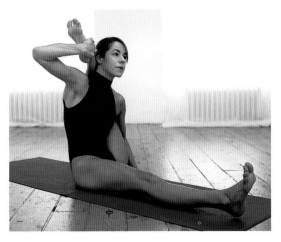

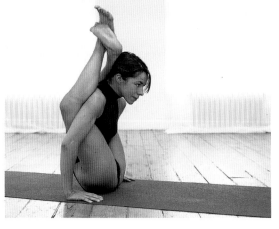

3 *Exhale*, softly rotate your left leg within its hip socket, and move your left knee back even more. Using your right hand, draw your left shin and ankle across behind your head and then your neck. Press your left side ribs forwards and lengthen up through your whole torso. Lift your face and press the back of your head backwards against your left ankle, drawing your chest up and shoulders wide to secure your left leg and foot in place.

4 *Inhale* and bend your right knee, drawing it deeply back, with your right hand, and up behind your right shoulder. With an *exhalation*, rotate your right knee outwards, and with your right hand again work your right shin and ankle behind your head and neck, crossing it over your left ankle. *Inhale* and place both hands on the floor on either side of your hips, lifting your chest and rolling your shoulders firmly back. This will help in taking the knees further back and securing your ankles in a crossed position behind your head. Press the back of your neck against your ankles and lift your face to look forwards.

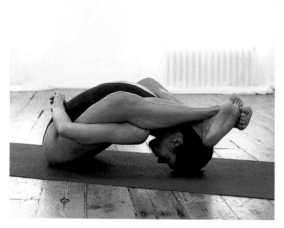

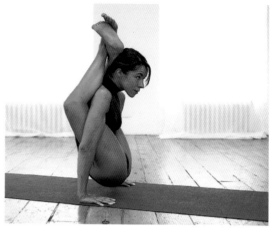

5 *Exhale*, step your hands forward and bend your elbows to lower your body forwards and down, placing your forehead on the floor. Thread your arms underneath your knees, turning your palms to face upwards and allowing your elbows to roll outwards. Now reach your hands back and clasp them together behind your waist. *Breathe five to ten full, deep breaths*, and gaze softly towards your third eye centre, <u>dristi</u>: **bhru madhya**.

Pratyahara
This sacred yogasana prepares us for pratyahara, or sensory withdrawal, which is the fifth limb of astanga yoga. Sensory withdrawal is symbolized here by the form of a tortoise drawing into its shell, moving attention away from the outer world and towards the inner life of the soul.

Easing into the pose
From step 1, rest your arms over your shinbones, bring the soles of your feet together and release your head forwards and down, so that your forehead is cradled in the arches of your feet. Once this is comfortable, progress on to slipping your arms under your knees and use a strap to link your hands. From here, enter your full vinyasa by raising your face and chest and placing your hands on the floor by the sides of your hips. Draw your feet in, crossing your ankles and tucking your knees up into your body to then jump back into Chaturanga Dandasana.

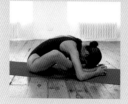 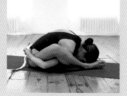

6 *Exhale*, release your hands and place them on the floor under your shoulders. Press down with your hands to raise your head and chest off the floor and so bring your torso upright. Straighten your arms with your ankles still strongly crossed behind your neck. As your torso rises, roll on to your buttocks and sit tall. *Inhale*, place your hands on the floor by the sides of your buttocks and lift your seat up off the floor as you press down through your arms and open your palms down into the ground. As you *breathe five steady breaths*, draw your chest open and move your shoulders and head back, looking forwards to your third eye centre, <u>dristi</u>: **bhru madhya**. After *five breaths*, *inhale*, uncross your ankles and stretch your legs into Tittibhasana. *Slowly exhale* as you fold your feet back into Bakasana and *inhale* here.

• On your next *exhalation*, softly jump your feet back into Chaturanga Dandasana and continue to flow into a **full vinyasa**. If you feel that the last five steps are too intense or strong at first, follow the instructions for easing into the posture.

Deepening the pose
This is a deep and intense posture, so work slowly and carefully into it, progressing gradually through the stages. As you place your forehead on the ground, gently extend your chin away from your chest and press your shoulders back to help prevent your feet from slipping forwards off the back of your head. When you have managed to catch hold of your hands, work towards deepening the bind by catching hold of the wrist, which will help to draw your shoulders further back and your chest and torso further forwards through your legs.

Garbha Piṇḍāsana A | WOMB EMBRYO POSTURE A

garbha = womb
pinda = embryo

Both Garbha Pindasanas and Kukkutasana are linked through breath and motion, one flowing into the other with no vinyasa. Garbha Pindasana A gently massages and tones the organs of the abdomen, particularly the liver.

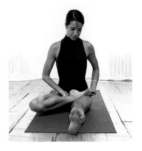 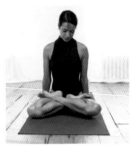 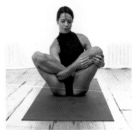 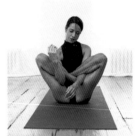

1 From Dandasana, *inhale very slowly*, bend your right knee and draw your right foot across on to the top of your left upper thigh into half lotus.

2 Continue to *inhale slowly* and bend your left knee, placing your left foot over on to your right upper thigh to come into the full lotus posture of Padmasana.

3 Still *inhaling*, draw your knees up and slide your right hand and forearm through the space between the front of your left ankle and the back of your right calf. Reach your hand along your left shinbone to feed your right elbow all the way through.

4 At the *end of your inhalation*, lift your right hand upwards to keep the right elbow in place, then slide your left hand and forearm through the gap between your right ankle and left calf. Slide your left forearm through until your left elbow is completely drawn through the gap.

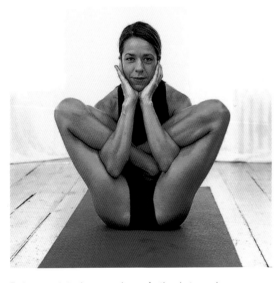

5 As you *exhale*, draw your knees further in towards your shoulders and bend both elbows strongly to lift your hands up under your chin and cradle your face, with your fingertips resting by your ears. Deepen your connection to uddiyana and mula bandha to help balance on your buttocks, and *take five to ten steady, deep breaths*, focusing forwards to your nose tip, <u>dristi</u>: **nasagrai**, before moving into Garbha Pindasana B.

Easing into the pose
If pain or strain is felt in your knees, proceed with caution and alternate the full lotus with a half lotus or with Sukhasana (cross-legged; see page 26). Wrap your arms around the outsides of your folded legs, clasping your hands around your ankles. To achieve the full posture, it may be useful to apply oil or

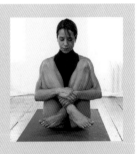

water to your hands up to your elbows to help your arms slip through your legs.

Deepening the pose
As your fingertips reach your ears, gently press the ears shut to withdraw your hearing. In this way, Garbha Pindasana furthers the preparation of pratyahara (the fifth limb of astanga yoga) as experienced in Supta Kurmasana, where you withdraw your focus from the external world in order to look within. Here, the finger pressure on your ears enables you to deepen your listening and to hear the internal sound of your breath alone.

Garbha Piṇḍāsana B and Kukkuṭāsana | WOMB EMBRYO POSTURE B AND ROOSTER POSTURE

garbha = womb
pinda = embryo
kukkuta = rooster

In Garbha Pindasana B, each roll of the soothing, rocking motion represents one of the nine months of gestation within the human womb. The lift of Kukkutasana develops strength in the upper body and especially in the wrists, arms and shoulders.

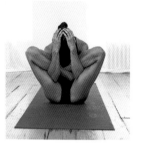
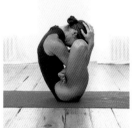
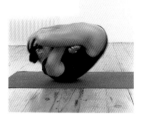
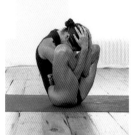

1a and b *Exhale* and move your chin in towards your chest, lowering your head and softly curling your body around like a ball. Place your palms on top of your head to seal yourself into this rounded shape.

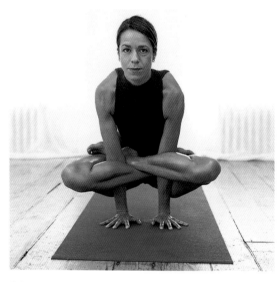

4 As you *inhale* into your ninth roll up, release your hands from your head and press your palms flat on to the floor with your fingers spreading open and pointing forwards. As your hands go down, press your chest strongly forwards and up. Lift the top of your head and firmly straighten your arms. As your arms straighten, raise your buttocks off the floor, connecting mula and uddiyana bandha deeper into your body. (Bandha control is exceptionally important here.) Balance on your broad, open hands and *take five to ten full, even breaths* here in Kukkutasana, looking towards your nose tip, <u>dristi</u>: **nasagrai**.

• *Exhale*, lower your seat to the floor and stretch into Dandasana. *Inhale*, draw your knees in and move into a **full vinyasa**.

2 As you continue to *exhale*, maintain the curve through your spine and softly roll back over on to your shoulders and swing your hips upwards.

3 *Inhale* and, as you begin to roll up, sway your hips slightly to the right side so that, as you arrive up on to your buttocks, you've rotated a little clockwise. *Exhale* and roll backwards again over your curved spine, and, as you begin to roll up with an *inhalation*, again sway your hips to the right so you rotate further clockwise. Repeat this rolling backwards and forwards in Garbha Pindasana another seven times (nine times in all) to complete a full circle.

Easing into the pose
As in the previous asana, you may wish to begin to practise this posture by wrapping your arms around the outside of your legs as you roll back and up. You can also build your strength towards the full balance by placing your hands on the ground by the sides of your hips to lift up

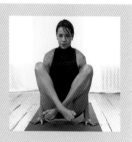

until you are able to slip your hands through your lotus legs.

Deepening the pose
Flow with the momentum of your breath to enhance a smooth, even, rolling motion and to connect yourself to the movement of your prana – the exhalation releasing your body down into the earth and the inhalation raising the energy of your body upwards.

Baddha Koṇāsana A/B | BOUND ANGLE POSTURE A/B

baddha = bound or caught
kona = angle

These postures free up energy within the pelvic region and allow it to flow down to the feet to improve blood circulation and power in the legs. The stretch forwards of the back refreshes and rejuvenates the kidneys, helping to allieviate urinary disorders.

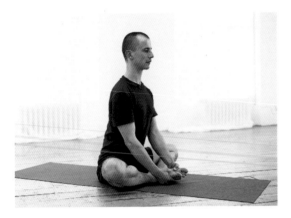

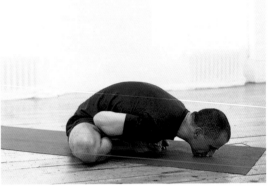

1 From Dandasana, *inhale*, bend your knees out to the sides and draw your feet together, bringing your heels close in towards your perineum and placing your hands on your feet. Now soften your hips and allow the soles of your feet to open upwards and the top of your feet to roll down into the floor. Open your inner thighs wide and draw your knees down evenly to the floor. Breathe length into your spine, lifting your chest up and lowering your chin down so that the back of your neck feels long. Gently slide your shoulders down and broaden through your collarbones as you *take five to ten slow, deep breaths*, looking towards your nose tip, <u>**dristi**</u>: **nasagrai**. On your last *inhalation*, lengthen still further through your back.

2 As you *exhale*, softly lengthen your back out and over the soles of your feet, hinging deeply in your hip sockets and sending your pubic bone backwards and down into the floor. Lengthen through the front of your spine, torso and throat to bring your chin on to the ground in front of your toes. Look towards your nose tip, <u>**dristi**</u>: **nasagrai**, and *breathe slowly and deeply* in Baddha Konasana A for *five to ten breaths*.

Easing into the pose

Sitting on a yoga block or firm cushion will help to give your spine a lift up and out of your hips. This can be especially helpful if you have tightness in your pelvis and it will help to prevent your lower back collapsing or rounding.

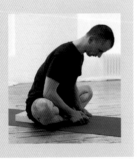

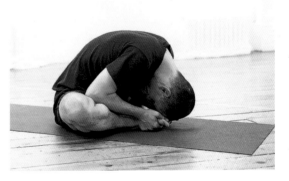

3 With an *inhalation*, return your torso upright and extend long through your back. On your *next exhalation*, deepen your engagement of uddiyana bandha to contract the abdomen in, softly curve your spine over and lower the top of your head down into the soles of your feet. Roll your chin inwards and release any tension in your shoulders by drawing your shoulder blades wide and down on either side of your spine. *Take five to ten deep, fluid breaths* in Baddha Konasana B while retaining your focus at the tip of your nose, <u>**dristi**</u>: **nasagrai**.

Deepening the pose

Tuck your elbows inwards on to your inner thighs, and, with each exhalation, gently apply pressure down on to your legs to encourage your hips to open, your inner thighs to release and your knees to descend.

• *Inhale*, draw your back up straight, and flow into a **full vinyasa**.

Upaviṣṭa Koṇāsana A | SEATED ANGLE POSTURE A

upavista = seated
kona = angle

This asana complements Baddha Konasana perfectly, as now the legs are stretched out, furthering the flow of energy from the pelvis to the feet. By releasing the legs wide and extending the torso forwards, flexibility in the hips and legs is developed.

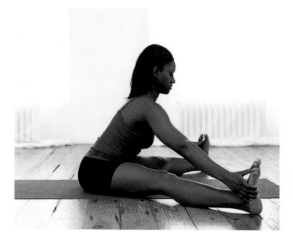

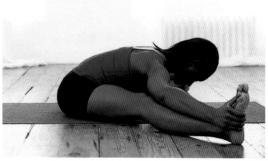

1 From landing in Dandasana from your **full vinyasa** continue to *inhale*, and stretch your legs open and wide out to the sides. Extend your back and lengthen through the front of your torso, stretching the abdominal wall long to tilt your pelvis forwards. Reach your hands on to your feet, placing each thumb in between the big toe and second toe joint and wrapping your fingers around the outer edges of your feet. Open your collarbones wide and press the centre of your chest forwards as you root your buttocks down into the floor, stretching both sides of your waist long.

2 On your *exhalation*, deepen the fold within your hips and pivot your pelvis forwards, sending your pubis and tailbone back and down behind you. Anchor your buttocks and backs of your legs firmly down into the floor. Open the centre of your chest forwards and out, lowering your torso towards the floor. Maintain uddiyana bandha and a long stretch through the front of your spine and throat to extend your chin towards the ground. Relax your shoulders and gently draw them back and down away from your ears. Focus awareness towards your third eye centre, **<u>dristi:</u> bru madhya**, and *take five to ten full, even breaths* here. As you breathe in this asana, with each *exhalation* soften in your hips and deepen uddiyana bandha as you release your torso long and further forwards and down. Now flow directly into Upavista Konasana B.

Easing into the pose
This posture develops flexibility in your hips, lower back and inner thighs. If these areas are tight, you may experience difficulty in reaching your hands to your feet. Rather than forcing the pose by rounding your back or bending your knees to catch hold of your feet, focus on creating full length and extension in both your

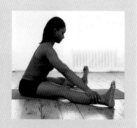

spine and legs, and place your hands on your ankles, or wherever you can manage, instead.

Deepening the pose
Engaging your bandhas in all postures is central to gaining internal support. In this asana, to extend deeper into the stretch without risk of groin strain, make sure you fully engage uddiyana and mula bandha to support the extension of your torso and the deep opening in your hips and thighs.

Be careful not to allow the front of your legs to roll inwards. Control this tendency by moving the outer edges of your thighs and knees backwards and down to direct your kneecaps and toes directly up. Keep your legs and feet active by extending your heels outwards and spreading your toes.

Upaviṣṭa Koṇāsana B | SEATED ANGLE POSTURE B

upavista = seated
kona = angle

Bandha control is essential here for providing support for the back when the torso is inclined and the legs extended up. As the body finds the balance point, the back and abdominal muscles are strengthened, helping to sustain alignment through the spine.

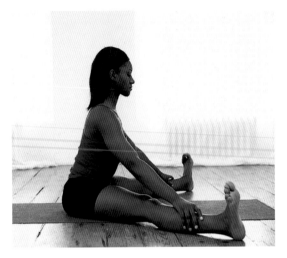

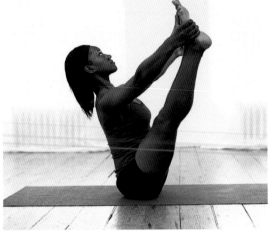

1 From Upavista Konasana A, *inhale* and lift your torso up while maintaining full length in your back and openness in your chest. Release the hand hold of your feet and slide your hands on to your shins.

2 As you continue to *inhale*, lift from uddiyana bandha and rock back on to your sitting bones while reclining your torso backwards. At the same time, lever your straight legs up and off the floor. As your feet float up, extend your hands to catch hold of the outer edge of your feet again (as in Upavista Konasana A). Now, lift and press your chest high and roll your shoulders softly back and down. Extend up and out of your lower back and stretch the sides of your waist long, raising your lower abdomen. Once balanced, send the fold in the front of your hips down into your sitting bones to stabilize yourself. As you *breathe five to ten full, steady breaths*, extend your legs longer with each breath and root your sitting bones into the floor to balance high upon them. Lift your face skywards and take your focus up to the third eye centre, <u>dristi</u>: **bru madhya**.

• After five to ten breaths, *exhale* and let go of your feet without allowing them to crash down. *Inhale*, bend your knees to cross your ankles, and press your hands into the floor to swing back into Chaturanga Dandasana and continue into a **full vinyasa**.

Easing into the pose
Keeping your back strong and straight is fundamental to achieving this asana. At first, therefore, it is more beneficial to bend your knees rather than risk collapsing in your spine and hunching your back. From a strong lifted spine and back, you can then work at gradually

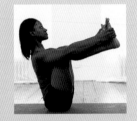

straightening your legs in this posture without shortening your torso.

Deepening the pose
Balancing high up on the tops of your sitting bones is the key to establishing a secure and open asana. Lifting from your lower back and bandhas while raising your chest strongly will help to shift your base forwards up on to your buttocks, rather then dropping back down on to your sacrum. It is a fine point of balance, and, once you're on it, you should continue to accentuate the lift through your chest by releasing your shoulders and stretching your legs like arrows.

Supta Koṇāsana A | SLEEPING ANGLE POSTURE A

97

SEATED ASANAS

supta = sleeping
kona = angle

As with all inverted postures the heart is placed on a higher level than the head. This stimulates the blood flow and oxygen supply to the brain. Sleeping angle posture introduces the first elements of inversion.

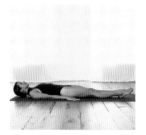
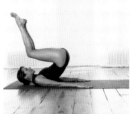
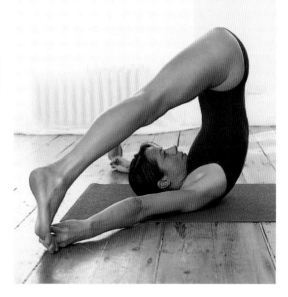

1 From Dandasana, *exhale* and softly roll your spine sequentially down on to the floor behind you, so that you are lying with your arms at the sides of your body, as if in a horizontal form of Tadasana.

2 *Inhale* and draw your knees up, pressing your arms and palms downwards as you swing your hips up and off the floor and roll over on to the back of your shoulders.

Benefits of the pose
Rolling on to the back of the neck releases the cervical vertebrae, stretching the muscles in this area to relieve stiffness and tension. The lifting of the pelvis intensifies the action and toning benefits of uddiyana bandha.

Easing into the pose
If this posture causes strain in your back, bend your knees slightly to get hold of your toes. Alternatively, if you experience difficulty holding your toes at first, hold your ankles while maintaining the stretch through your legs, then gradually move towards your toes.

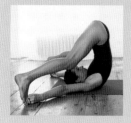
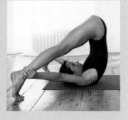

3 As you *exhale*, continue to roll completely over on to the back of your neck and head. Take your feet overhead and part them wide, stretching your inner thighs open. Catch hold of your right big toe with your right index and middle fingers and your left big toe with your left index and middle fingers. Press your sitting bones and pubis upwards to draw length into the front and back of your spine, and lock your chest up and into your chin. Extend your heels away, with your toes tucked under, and feel the stretch through the entire length of the back of your legs. *Take five to ten deep, long breaths*, focusing towards your nose tip, **dristi: nasagrai**, and deeply engage your bandhas to prepare for Supta Konasana B, which flows directly on from here.

Deepening the pose
To enter this asana from step 1, as your back and abdominal muscles develop strength, try lifting your legs up straight and together and then rolling over on to the back of your shoulders. While in this posture, focus on opening the back of your neck and shoulders wide into the floor, at the same time as raising your pelvis higher to feel the polarity of energy directions through your body.

Supta Koṇāsana B | SLEEPING ANGLE POSTURE B

supta = sleeping
kona = angle

The motion of rolling up through the spine helps to align the vertebrae and massages the back muscles along the floor. The head gently swinging up and down boosts the blood circulation from the brain to the heart, clearing the mind and refreshing the body.

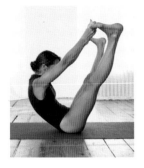 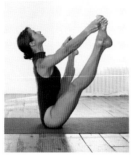

1 From Supta Konasana A, *inhale* and press from your tucked-under toes, gently rounding your back like a ball to roll up sequentially through your spine. Maintain your finger hold of your big toes, and send the top of your head forwards in order to roll smoothly upwards.

2 At the top of your *inhalation*, and just as you roll up on to your buttocks, strongly lift your chest forwards and up. Softly throw your shoulders back and extend through your spine to move your back from a curved to a straight position. Send the fold in the front of your hips down into your sitting bones to stabilize yourself here, and take a moment to suspend yourself in this fine point of balance, lifting your face and heart skywards as you look to your third eye centre, **dristi: bru madhya**.

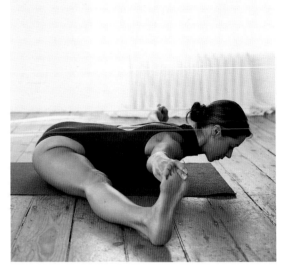

3 As you *exhale*, drop forwards into Upavista Konasana, flexing your legs and feet fully and strongly with your fingers still securely holding your toes. This will carry the whole shape of the previous suspended position down on to the floor. Slide your shoulder blades down your back and lengthen the front of your torso along the floor, moving your chest forwards and your chin down towards the ground. On your next *inhalation*, and while still holding your toes, lift your body upwards, drawing more openness into your chest. With an *exhalation*, release your hands from your feet and bring your torso completely upright.

• *Inhale*, cross your ankles and press your hands into the floor to lift your seat up. Swing your feet back into Chaturanga Dandasana and continue to flow into a **full vinyasa** to softly land into Dandasana.

Easing into the pose

This flowing, rolling motion up and then down takes practice to achieve, and careful attention to how you roll through your back and drop forwards is essential. Keeping your back and spine consciously rounded will help you to roll like a ball, and, if keeping your legs totally straight impedes your sense of momentum at first, try bending them slightly as you roll upwards. However, once you reach your point of balance, stretch your legs long and your back straight. As you drop forwards, be careful not to crash land on your heels, though this may prove difficult, especially if, in the beginning, your tendency is to bend your knees. If this is the case, place your feet down one at a time until your flexibility and strength have developed sufficiently for you to progress on to the straight-leg drop forwards, as discussed in the "Deepening the pose" box (*right*).

Deepening the pose

Focus on completely flexing your feet and stretching your legs straight, so that as you drop forwards your heels do not touch the floor. This will not only develop both strength and flexibility in your legs but will also ensure that your calf muscles cushion your landing into Upavista Konasana B, rather than letting your heels crash down. Your bandhas, too, will greatly help a soft landing, so consciously engage them into your body and allow your body to flow and roll with the natural momentum of your breath.

Supta Pādāṅguṣṭhāsana | SLEEPING FOOT BIG TOE POSTURE

supta = sleeping
pada = foot or leg
angustha = big toe

The preceding postures have prepared the muscles of the legs for the deep stretch of this pose. As one leg is lengthened up and over into the torso to increase flexibility, the other presses down and along the floor in the opposite direction to develop strength.

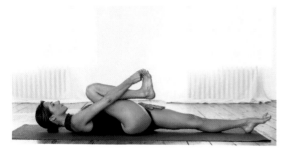

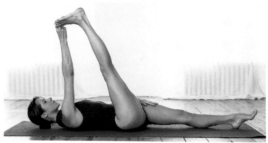

1 *Exhale* from Dandasana and softly roll your back sequentially on to the floor to lay your body long and straight. In this supine position, *inhale*, draw your right thigh and knee up, folding deeply within your right hip socket, and catch hold of your right big toe with your right index and middle fingers. Extend your left leg long, pressing the left sole of your foot out and away from your hips.

2 At the end of your *inhalation*, straighten your right leg completely by extending your right foot up and anchoring down through the back of your right hip to maintain even alignment through your pelvis. Lengthen through your back and broaden your shoulders and sacrum into the floor. Press your left palm firmly down on to your left thigh to encourage the full extension of your left leg.

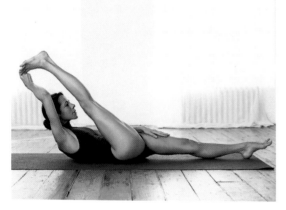

Easing into the pose
If you are unable to hold your big toe with your leg straight, take a strap and wrap it around the ball of your lifted foot. Work in this way until you are flexible enough to catch hold of your toe. If you have suffered from a back injury or any back pain, practise by bending your lifted leg and hugging your knee in with both hands as you lift your head and shoulders. This will help to develop abdominal strength and realign your spine. As you get stronger, work the full asana.

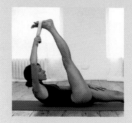
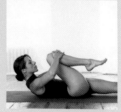

3 As you *exhale*, deepen the connection of uddiyana bandha into your body and raise your head, shoulders and upper back off the floor, moving your right leg up and in towards your face. Stretch out through your left leg, pressing your left heel and ball of the foot away and opening the entire length of the back of your left leg down into the floor. This creates a strong base for the stretching of your right leg. Be careful not to hunch your shoulders; instead, let them open wide and bend your right elbow sideways as your head draws higher towards your right leg. *Take five to ten steady, deep breaths* in this asana, looking towards the toes of your right foot, <u>dristi</u>: **padhayoragrai**. After a minimum of five breaths, *inhale* and, with control, softly lower your head, shoulders and upper back down on to the floor, as in step 2. From here, move directly into the next asana.

Deepening the pose
Keep both legs and torso evenly active – not overstretching or overworking one side of your body while the other side is underactive. Stretch the back of your lifted leg long and press the back of both hips evenly into the floor. Deeply activate uddiyana bandha by flattening the abdominal wall down as you move your chin to your shin.

Supta Pārśvasahita A | SLEEPING SIDE ACCOMPANIED POSTURE A

supta = sleeping
parsva = side or lateral
sahita = accompanied

As the lifted leg is opened out to the side, the stretch through the leg muscles is intensified and a balance between flexibility and strength is developed. The lifting and rotation of the leg also promotes full blood circulation through the legs into the feet.

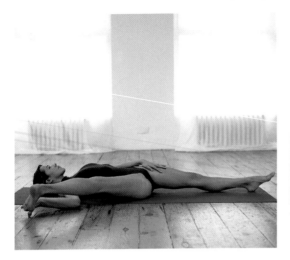

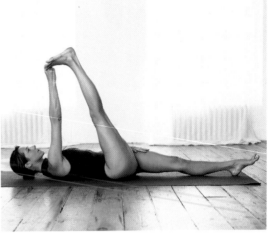

1 From Supta Padangusthasana, maintaining your finger hold of your right big toe, *slowly exhale* and rotate your right leg, deep within its hip socket, outwards to the right side. Fully engage uddiyana bandha to stabilize the pelvis into the floor. Open and stretch both your right arm and leg wide, lengthening through your right inner thigh until your right toes make contact with the floor. Press your left shoulder, left side of your ribcage, left buttock and the back of your left leg firmly down into the floor to create a strong, secure foundation from which to release and open your right leg out. This gives balance and stability to the stretch of your body in this asana. *Breathe five to ten full, even breaths*, take your focus towards the left, **dristi**: **parsva**.

2 *Inhale*, draw your right leg up from the right side and anchor down through the back of your right hip while extending your right foot high and your leg long. Spread your back wide and open into the floor before continuing directly into Supta Parsvasahita B.

Easing into the pose
If you have been working with a strap in the previous posture, continue to do so for this asana. Alternatively, if you practised the previous pose with your knee bent, continue to do so, and open your bent leg out to the side with your hand cupping and supporting your knee.

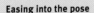

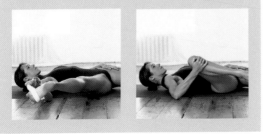

Deepening the pose
As in all of our asanas, both sides of the body need to work equally for strength and flexibility. Particularly in this posture, any imbalances of strength and flexibility through the right and left side become very apparent. It is therefore important to feel that both sides of your body are consciously involved and aware. Focus to open the left side of your body deeply into the floor away from your right side, as your right leg opens out and away from your left side.

If you find the left side of your body losing contact with the floor as your right leg opens to the side, this is an indication of imbalance between your strength and flexibility. To address this imbalance, move your right leg up to reanchor your left side down, and stabilize the pose here. From this centred place, focus on slowly releasing your right leg out and your left side down while maintaining full contact with the floor through the left side of your back. In this way, balance is created and flexibility and strength developed together, rather than one at the expense of the other.

Supta Pārśvasahita B | SLEEPING SIDE ACCOMPANIED POSTURE B

supta = sleeping
parsva = side or lateral
sahita = accompanied

This posture is an intensified form of Supta Padangusthasana and is considered a purifying asana, as the deep and dynamic articulation of the legs focuses and stills the mind, helping to harness sexual energy.

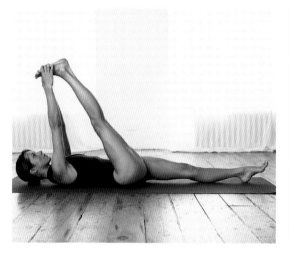

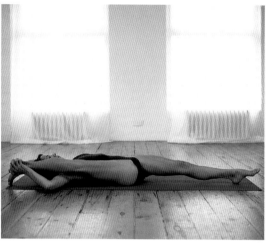

1 From Supta Parsvasahita A, with an *exhalation* take both your hands to catch hold of your right foot. Level your shoulders and draw the whole surface of your back and the back of your pelvis open and down into the floor. Press the heel and ball of your left foot away.

2 Continue to *exhale* and bend your elbows wide, keeping your chest open and both shoulders releasing down into the floor, and draw your right leg straight over to the right side of your head. Extend your right toes to touch the floor. Holding your foot with both hands still, bring your right inner calf to touch softly against your right ear and engage uddiyana bandha. *Breathe five to ten deep, even breaths,* looking to your nose tip, <u>dristi</u>: **nasagrai**. Focus on softening deeply in your right hip and through the back of your right thigh to extend and release into the posture fully. *Inhale* and return your leg to upright (at a right angle to your left leg), remaining open in your shoulders and centred in your back. *Exhale* and let go of your right foot, slowly releasing your right leg straight down to the floor by the side of your left leg to lie in a supine Tadasana. Without a vinyasa, repeat Supta Padangusthasana and Supta Parsvasahita A and B on the left side, then move into Chakrasana, as overleaf.

Easing into the pose
If you have been using a strap in the two previous postures, you will need to continue to do so. Do not, however, attempt to draw your leg beyond 90 degrees to the floor until you are able to catch hold of your foot while maintaining full length and straightness in both legs. A softer option

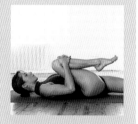

would be to hug your thigh in towards your front torso as you bend your knee.

Deepening the pose
As with Supta Padangusthasana and Supta Parsvasahita A, working evenly in this asana is essential for establishing balance in your body. In this pose it is easy to forget about engaging your bandhas and stretching your left leg while overfocusing on the lifting of your right leg in the ambition to deepen the stretch of this asana. Instead, draw your awareness into your left leg, opening the back of your knee down into the ground and extending your foot away from your hips. Engaging your bandhas will help to support your back, keep your torso long and your chest open as your body releases into this deep and demanding posture.

Chakrāsana | CIRCLING WHEEL POSTURE

chakra = circle or wheel

The circular wheeling momentum of the body in this transitional posture boosts the circulation through the spine to the brain, as the back muscles are rolled and massaged into the floor to refresh and awaken the complete body.

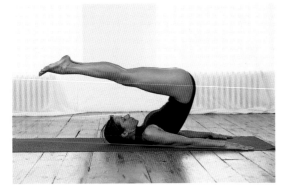

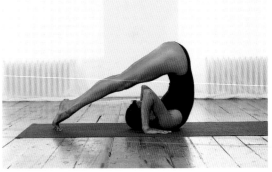

1 *Inhale*, draw your knees up, and press your arms and palms down by the sides of your body to help swing your hips and pelvis gently up off the floor. As your hips rise, soften your spine round, rolling further up and over your back on to your shoulders, like a ball rolling backwards. Let your pelvis float and the back of your neck and shoulders release wide and down into the floor.

2 Continue to *inhale*. Lengthen your legs, reaching your feet overhead, on to the floor. Take your hands on to the floor by the sides of your head. Your fingertips must be just under your shoulders with your elbows bent and pointing directly upwards.

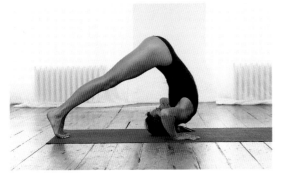

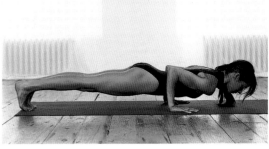

3 Towards the *end of your inhalation*, roll over on to the back of your head, allowing your neck to stretch gently with the rest of your spine rolling up off the floor. Press firmly down through your palms and stretch your legs strongly, with your toes tucked under. Transfer your weight now fully on to your hands and feet to roll further over on to the back and top of your head.

4 *Exhale* as you deepen uddiyana bandha, feeling dynamic energy pouring into your arms and legs. Release your head forwards and out to complete this full circular motion of Chakrasana and softly pounce out into Chaturanga Dandasana.

• From here, flow through a **full vinyasa**.

Easing into the pose
Go slowly, practising just up to step 2, gradually building your confidence to go further each time. Resist the tendency to roll over on to one shoulder more than the other by pressing evenly into both hands. Keep your mind relaxed and let it flow with the roll.

Deepening the pose
At all times it is of prime importance to keep your neck relaxed and your bandhas engaged, as this will enable you to roll with ease and without panic over your shoulders and neck. Be aware here of jalandhara bandha and allow your throat to yield.

Ubhaya Pādāṅguṣṭhāsana | BOTH FEET BIG TOE POSTURE

ubhaya = both
pada = foot or leg
angustha = big toe

The soft, rolling motion of the preceding postures continues in the next two asanas, stimulating the spine and back muscles and helping to prepare for the back bends that follow. Ubhaya Padangusthasana also strengthens the back and tones the legs.

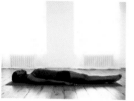
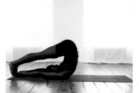

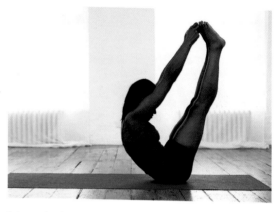

1 From Dandasana, *exhale* and roll your back down sequentially to lie supine on the floor.

2 *Inhale*, drawing your knees up and press your arms and hands down by the sides of your body. Roll your hips up, softly curling through your back to roll over on to the back of your shoulders. Extend your feet overhead, stretching your legs long with your inner thighs and feet together. Reach your hands to your feet to catch hold of your big toes with your index and middle fingers. *Exhale* here and soften the back of your neck. Release your shoulders wide into the floor as you draw your hips further over your shoulders and press your heels away.

3 As you begin to *inhale*, push off from your tucked-under toes. Deepen uddiyana bandha. Softly round your back, keeping your chin resting on your chest, and roll up through the curl of your spine. Lengthen the backs of your legs and lead the crown of your head forwards.

Easing into the pose
To gain a sense of momentum in this posture, practise rolling backwards and forwards with a curved spine and the knees slightly bent. Once you find a balance on your buttocks, work your back straight first and then your legs. If your back rounds as your legs straighten, rebend your knees to re-establish length through your spine, then try

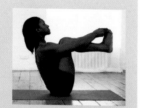

again to lengthen your legs while maintaining the straightness of your spine. Do not straighten your legs at the expense of rounding your back.

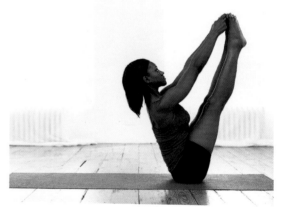

4 Continue to *inhale* as your sitting bones make contact with the floor. Strongly project your chest open and upwards, lifting your heart high and face skywards. Release your shoulders back and lengthen your back out of its curve, balancing high up on your sitting bones. Deepen uddiyana bandha and stretch your legs as far as possible, looking towards your third eye centre, <u>dristi</u>: **bru madhya**, as you *take five full breaths*.

Deepening the pose
This posture is again a fine point of balance, and instead of passing through it, as in Supta Konasana, we maintain and breathe into it. To feel the correct placement up on your sitting bones and not collapse into your sacrum, send the fold at the front of your hips down into your sitting bones and lift strongly up from your lower back, pressing the sacrum and back of your waist forwards. Then release your neck and head back, stretching through the front of your throat.

• *Exhale*, and release the clasp of your toes, placing your hands on the floor by your hips and bending your knees to cross your ankles. As you take your next *inhalation*, press down through your arms and raise your seat to enter into a **full vinyasa**.

Ūrdhva Mukha Paschimottānāsana
UPWARD FACING INTENSE STRETCH OF THE WEST POSTURE

urdhva = upward
mukha = face
paschima = west
uttana = intense stretch

This is a progression from Ubhaya Padangusthasana, and the benefits are intensified by the pressure of the length of the front torso into the legs. This stretches and tones the abdominal wall, increasing the blood flow around and through the internal organs.

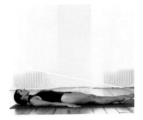 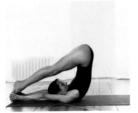 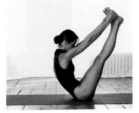 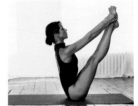

1 Landing in Dandasana from a full vinyasa, continue to *inhale* and roll your back sequentially down to lie supine on the floor. Keep *inhaling* now as you roll your hips up, softly curling through your back to roll over on to the back of your shoulders.

2 Complete your *inhalation* and extend your feet overhead, stretching your legs long with your inner thighs and feet together. Reach your hands to your feet to catch hold of their outer edge. *Exhale*, maintaining the hold of your feet, soften the back of your neck and release your shoulders wide as you draw your hips further up and press your heels away.

3 Push from your tucked-under toes and, as you *inhale,* softly round your back by deepening uddiyana bandha. Keep your chin resting into your chest to roll up through the curve of your spine like a ball rolling forwards. Lengthen the backs of your legs as you send the top of your head forwards.

4 Continue to *inhale* and, as your sitting bones make contact with the floor, strongly project your chest open and up, lift your head, aligning your neck with your spine, and extend your focus up to your toes, <u>dristi</u>: **padhayoragrai**. Release your shoulders back and lengthen your back out of its curve, securing your balance high up on your sitting bones. Deepen uddiyana bandha and stretch your legs as far as possible.

5 *Exhale* and release the hold of your feet, then recatch them, interlacing your fingers around the balls of your feet, or taking your right hand to hold your left wrist. Lengthen up through the front of your spine and torso, raising your chest and sending your pubic bone downwards. Lift out of your sacrum and stretch your back, bending your elbows to draw your legs and torso together. Draw your legs in towards your front torso and your torso in towards your legs. *Take five to ten long, steady breaths*, focusing energy up to your toes, <u>dristi</u>: **padhayoragrai**. *Inhale* and draw your torso and legs away from one another, still holding your feet. *Exhale* and release your feet. Bend your knees to cross your ankles, with your hands on the floor by your hips.

• *Inhale*, press down through your palms and lift your hips, then move into a **full vinyasa**, to jump through into Dandasana.

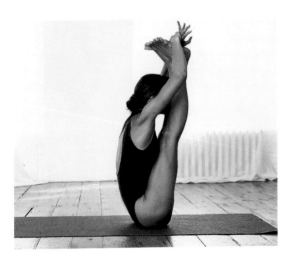

Easing into the pose
If drawing your legs and torso together causes your back to round or collapse, practise only up to step 4.

Deepening the pose
As you become stronger and more supple, focus on moving your chin and forehead up along your shinbones as you slide your shoulder blades down your back. Fold deeply in your hips to draw your legs and torso together like the pages of a book shutting.

Setu Bandhāsana | BRIDGE POSTURE

setu = bridge
bandha = bondage or fetter

In this posture, an arching bridge shape is created through the body, producing spinal flexibility and preparing the back muscles for the back bend of Urdhva Dhanurasana. This pose strengthens the neck, dorsal, lumbar, sacral and back thigh muscles.

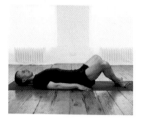

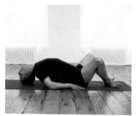

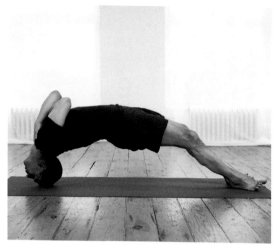

1 From Dandasana, *exhale* and roll sequentially down your spine to lie on your back. Now bend your knees, allowing them to part wide while turning your feet out and placing your heels together but your big toes apart. Open the soles of your feet face down towards the floor and place your arms by the sides of your body with your palms pressing down.

2 As you begin to *inhale*, arch through your spine, lifting your chest up and stretching through the front of your neck. Draw the very top of your head on to the floor. Tilt your pelvis, pressing your sitting bones down and raising the back of your waist and your ribs up. Spread your feet and toes while relaxing your face as you look towards your nose tip.

3 Continue to *inhale*, rooting down through your feet, and send your hips up, raising your seat off the floor. As your hips lift higher, press your feet into the ground to straighten your legs and arch deeper through your upper spine, opening up your chest. Be careful not to grip your buttocks, as they will automatically engage and, if you overclench them, this will block the lift of your pelvis and lower spine. Release your hands from the floor and cross your arms over your chest. *Take five deep, smooth breaths* and look towards your nose tip, <u>dristi</u>: **nasagrai**. *Exhale* to lower your buttocks down. Release off the top of your head and lie your back flat on the floor, placing your arms at your sides.

• From here, lift your legs and roll back into Chakrasana and move into a **full vinyasa**. Jump through to land in Dandasana.

Benefits of the pose
Setu Bandha is a wonderful tonic for the entire body. The expansion of the chest and front ribs opens the heart to stimulate circulation and increases lung capacity.

Easing into the pose
If this posture is too strong on your neck and creates pressure, take your hands back on to the floor by the sides of your head with your fingertips pointing towards your feet. Press your palms down and roll your shoulders back to draw your chest open and high. Alternatively,

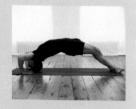

if you find this too intense, practise the back bend moderation of Urdhva Dhanurasana overleaf.

Deepening the pose
In this asana in order not to compress your neck vertebrae the legs must be fully active and the bandhas deeply engaged. As you practise this asana, concentrate on standing your feet firmly on the floor as you lift your kneecaps, thighs and abdominal muscles upwards. Draw your spine, especially your upper spine, up and in, pressing it through into the front of your torso to help raise your chest and ease pressure out of your neck.

Ūrdhva Dhanurāsana | UPWARD BOW POSTURE

urdhva = upward
dhanu = bow

This strong back bend provides the body with a counter-stretch to the earlier forward bending postures. The front of the abdomen, hips and thighs are fully stretched and lengthened, and the hands and wrists are strengthened.

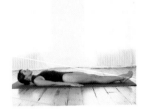

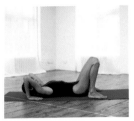

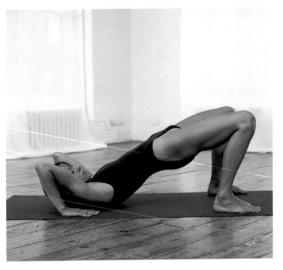

1 From Dandasana, begin to *exhale* and softly roll your back down to lie straight and flat on the floor, arms by your sides.

2 Continue to *exhale*, bending your knees and stepping your feet parallel and in line with the outer edge of your hips. Move your heels in so they touch the outer edge of your buttocks. Place your palms down on the floor on either side of your head, in line with your shoulders. Open your hands and extend your fingers underneath the tops of your shoulders, and direct your elbows upwards.

3 As you begin to *inhale*, press the soles of your feet into the floor, move your hips upwards and fully engage uddiyana bandha to support your lower back. Maintain the parallel alignment of your feet and legs as you move on to the next step.

Easing into the pose
Back bends are known for invigorating the nervous system and relieving nervousness, anxiety and fear. However, if a full back bend feels too intense, refer to the Urdhva Dhanurasana moderations.

Deepening the pose
As you gain in strength, suppleness and stamina, instead of lowering your whole body down to the floor, just bend your elbows to lower the top of your head to touch the ground as you exhale. From here, with your head still on the floor, take a step with each hand in towards your feet. Then, with a full inhalation, press firmly and evenly into your hands and feet to straighten your arms and energize your legs, raising your

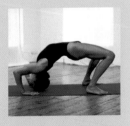

chest, torso and pelvis into a higher arch still. Take five steady breaths and repeat the lowering down on to your head and stretching back up twice more before releasing out of the asana.

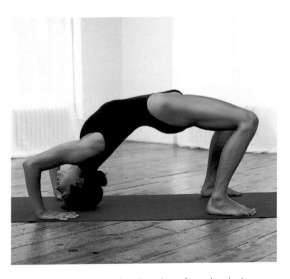

4 Continue to *inhale*, pressing the palms of your hands down and lifting your shoulders up off the floor. Open your chest to place the top of your head on the ground, and begin to arch in your upper back. Transfer all your weight evenly through your arms and legs. Engage uddiyana bandha to lengthen through the abdominal wall and give support to your lower back.

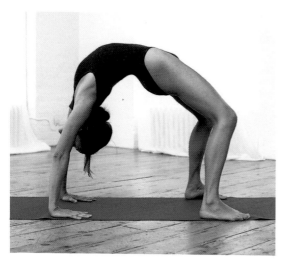

5 As you complete your *inhalation*, send energy down through your arms and legs into your hands and feet and press them firmly and evenly into the floor. Stretch your arms straight and roll your shoulders back, away from your ears, sending your shoulder blades into your back ribs. Do not tense your buttocks, as this will block movement in your lower spine. Draw your thigh muscles up to raise your hips, torso and chest higher. Slide your tailbone in towards your pubis. Feel the front of your pelvis opening: this will help you to arch evenly through the entire length of your spine. *Take five to ten deep breaths*, looking towards your nose tip, **dristi: nasagrai**. Then *exhale* and bend your elbows and knees, softly lowering your back on to the floor to the position shown in step 2. Repeat steps 3–5 twice more, so that you practise this asana three times in all, taking your body a little deeper into the posture with each repetition.

• Then, with an *inhalation*, roll over into Chakrasana to move into a **full vinyasa** landing on your feet into Tadasana.

Ūrdhva Dhanurāsana moderated | UPWARD BOW POSTURE MODERATED

This moderated posture can be practised initially to build the strength and flexibility necessary for the back bends of Setu Bandha and Urdhva Dhanurasana. It is a gentler asana than the full postures, with extra support provided from the base of the neck, head and arms as they press and root downwards, helping to arch the spine upwards.

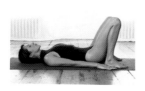

1 Follow steps 1 and 2 of Urdhva Dhanurasana, but instead of putting your hands beside your head, keep your arms at the side of your body with your palms facing down.

Easing into the pose
If you are unable to interlace your fingers while maintaining contact with your little fingers into the floor, leave your arms straight by your sides and press the entire length of them down, rolling your elbows in towards each other.

Deepening the pose
As the arch develops through your back and your legs grow stronger, try stepping your feet inwards so that you can clasp your ankles securely. Extend your heels down to send your hips higher, and draw your knees

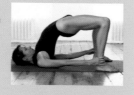

completely over and in line with your ankles.

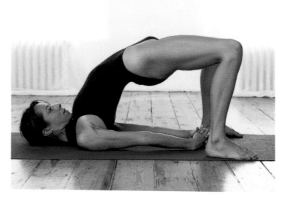

2 *Inhale*, press firmly down through the soles of your feet into the floor, and raise your pelvis high without clenching your buttock muscles. Interlace your fingers on the floor behind your back, rolling your shoulders down and away from your ears and lengthening your arms. Extend your elbows, wrists and little fingers into the floor, moving your spine and back ribs in and up. Open up your chest, lifting it in towards your chin, and relax your throat and jaw. *Take five to ten even breaths*, gently drawing your tailbone in towards your pubis, still without clenching your buttocks. Focus on developing the support from the strength in your legs by extending your feet down and lifting your thigh muscles up, helping to raise your pelvis higher and to arch deeply through your spine.

Ūrdhva Dhanurāsana drop back | UPWARD BOW POSTURE DROP BACK

The rooting down through the feet into the floor is absolutely essential and provides the foundation of this sequence. The free-flowing motion of the spine cascading backwards not only invigorates the entire body and mind but also helps to combat fear and develop trust and self-confidence.

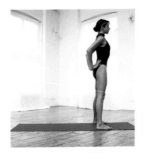
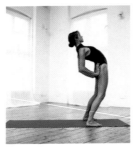
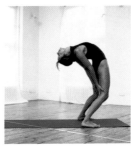
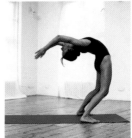

1 From **Tadasana**, *inhale* and jump your feet apart into a parallel position slightly wider than your hips. Breathe length into your spine and root firmly down through your feet, placing your hands on the back of your pelvis. Draw your shoulders open and lift your chest, looking straight ahead.

2 As you begin to *exhale*, move your tailbone in and down and press your sacrum forwards, drawing your pelvis over your toes. Use the pressure of your hands to help sway your whole pelvis forwards. Engage uddiyana bandha, lengthening through your abdomen and lifting up and out from your lower back. Open your chest and strongly roll your shoulders back. Now stretch your spine up and curve through your upper back, anchoring securely down through your legs into your feet. Root your feet deeply into the floor.

3 Continue to *exhale*, arching further back, and press your sacrum and pelvis strongly forwards as you release your head, shoulders and chest backwards. Stretch your arms back, taking your palms on to the backs of your legs, and arch deeply through the length of your spine to release your head back.

4 Continue to *exhale*, release your hands rotating your arms overhead and bring your palms together. Draw your head further back to arch deeper still and look to the floor behind your heels.

Easing into the pose

This backward cascade should be learnt with a teacher, who will be able to support and guide you. Once you have been guided through this sequence, you may wish to try it alone. A safe way to do this is to place a few cushions on the floor against the wall. Stand about 60cm/2ft away from the wall and arch your spine back, taking your hands on to the wall. Then slowly walk your hands down the wall on to the floor. Once your hands are on the ground, arch into Urdhva Dhanurasana. Walk your hands up the wall to stand upright.

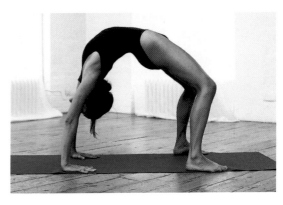

5 *Exhale* completely while maintaining a strong lift through your thighs, abdomen and chest to drop your fingertips then palms down on to the floor, and, with a springy motion through your elbows, stretch your arms straight as your hands land to prevent your head dropping on to the floor. *Inhale* and rock your weight over on to your hands and then forwards on to your feet. As you shift your weight on to your feet, push off from your palms and fingers into a rebounding action leading up through your pelvis to swing your hips forwards and then your entire torso to stand vertically. Take your palms together in front of your chest and then replace your hands on your hips. With your next *exhalation*, cascade your body backwards and down again into **Urdhva Dhanurasana**, and with an *inhalation*, swing back up to stand again. Practise this drop-back three times.

Deepening the pose

Once you become more confident in this liberating cascade backwards, start with your hands in the prayer position (namaste) at the centre of your chest, and, as you begin to arch through your spine, stretch your arms directly over your head to let your hands lead the way back and down on to the floor.

Adho Mukha Vṛkṣāsana | DOWNWARD FACING TREE POSTURE

adho = downward
mukha = face
vrksa = tree

This posture builds strength in the hands, wrists, arms and shoulders. The jump up into the hand balance is a development of the jump through of the vinyasa, so the same principle of swinging the pelvis up to align over the shoulders and wrists applies.

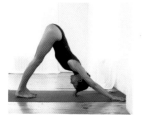
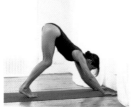

1 Begin in Adho Mukha Svanasana, with your fingers 1cm/½in away from the wall. Open your palms securely into the floor, as your hands are now going to be your foundation. Broaden across your shoulders, connect your arms into their sockets.

2 *Exhale* and bend your knees softly, releasing a little weight back on to your feet, preparing to pounce upwards from your toes.

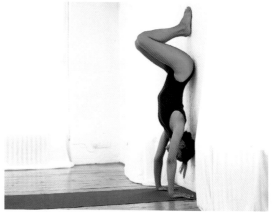

3 *Inhale* and lifting from uddiyana bandha jump strongly from your feet. Swing your hips in a high arch up and over your shoulders to shift your weight completely on to your hands. Bring the back of your pelvis and the soles of your feet on to the wall. Stretch your arms straight, pressing your palms down.

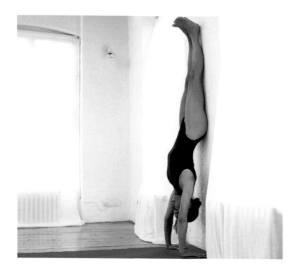

4 *Exhale* and extend your legs long, drawing your heels and inner thighs together. Lengthen through your waist and back, and *breathe five to ten full, steady breaths*, looking towards your nose tip, <u>dristi</u>: nasagrai.

Easing into the pose
To get the full lift of your hips up and over your shoulders, it may help at first to swing one leg up and then the other. From Adho Mukha Svanasana, step one foot forwards, look to the space between your hands and raise uddiyana bandha into your body. Then swing 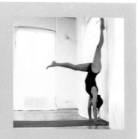 one leg up and over, followed by the other.

Finishing the seated postures
This sequence of postures is closed by the forward bend of Paschimottanasana which is the first asana of our seated series and forms the ultimate counter-stretch and release from the preceding back bends. Followed by a full vinyasa, this creates a full circle by finishing where we began.

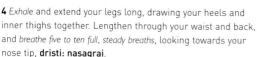

Deepening the pose
Practise the feeling of a free-standing hand balance by moving the top of your head forwards to rest on the wall, then release the feet from the wall, using the contact of your head against the wall to steady you. Take care not to overarch. Deeply engage uddiyana bandha 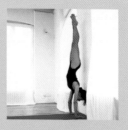 and draw your spine long, extending up to your feet.

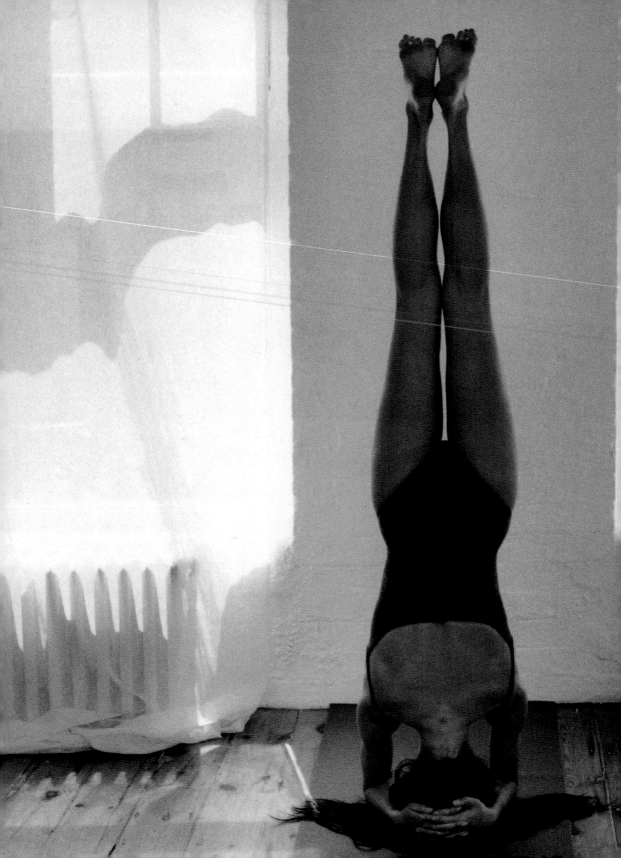

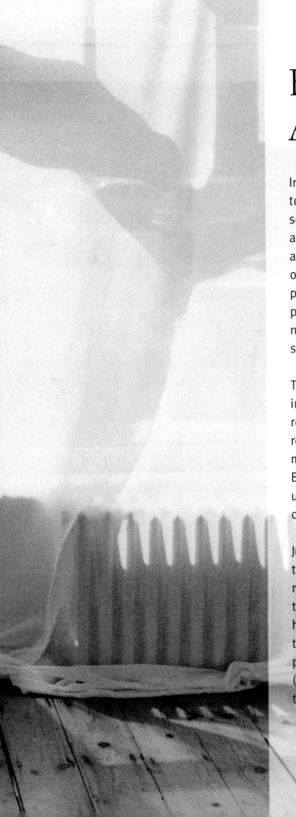

Finishing Asanas

In the finishing postures we turn upside down to practise the shoulder and headstand sequences. Turning upside down can induce a sense of disorientation, insecurity, fear and anxiety, so challenging our comfortable view of the world. But if we practise with gentle patience and calmness, these inverted postures help us to clear our mind of negativity and find our own internal balance, security and stability.

The feet, which have been so firmly rooted into the earth, are now released skywards and root into the heavens instead, symbolically removing our standing in the physical and material world to seek inspiration from above. Bringing the head on to the floor to balance upon it helps to focus the mind, surrendering our thoughts to the earth and ground.

Just as Surya Namaskara reflects the energy of the sun, warming the body and awakening the mind, this finishing sequence is reflective of the moon's energy. It balances the body and harmonizes the mind, preparing the way for the meditative posture of Padmasana (lotus posture) and the deep relaxation of Savasana (corpse posture), which is the final pose of the primary series.

Sālamba Sarvāngāsana | SUPPORTED WHOLE BODY POSTURE

salamba = supported
sarva = entire or whole
anga = limb or body

Sarvangasana is the mother posture, creating harmony and balance throughout the human system. The inversion of the body boosts the circulatory and respiratory systems, and so nourishes and revitalizes the entire body on a cellular level.

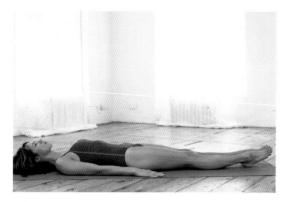

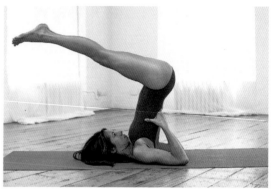

1 From a full vinyasa, *inhale* and jump through to land in Dandasana. *Exhale* and softly roll sequentially down through your spine to lie supine and straight on the floor, with your arms close by your sides. Feel the back surface of your body long against the floor and soften your shoulders down into the ground as you *take five full breaths.*

2 *Inhale,* pressing the back of your shoulders, arms and palms down into the floor, then draw your legs up and roll over on to the back of your shoulders and neck. Engage uddiyana bandha to create a lift through your pelvis and torso as you raise your hips directly over and in line with your shoulders. Move your chest up and into your chin, bending your elbows inwards no further apart than the width of your shoulders, and place your palms firmly on your back.

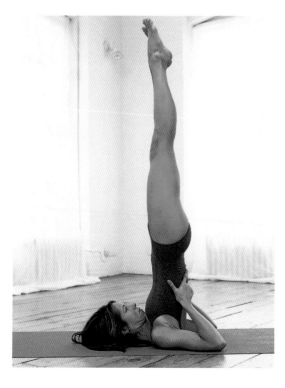

3 Continue to *inhale*, and stretch your legs up straight, coming into the full posture of Salamba Sarvangasana, balancing your entire body up and over on to the very top of your shoulders and back of your neck and head. Lift up out of your neck and shoulders by taking your hands lower down and pressing your palms on to your back ribs to help draw your upper spine away from your neck. Lengthen through your legs, opening the soles of your feet skywards, and align your heels together, directly up and over your hips. Move your tailbone in towards your pubic bone and draw your thigh muscles up and on to their thighbones. Draw in your lower abdomen to deepen uddiyana bandha. *Breathe here for 20–30 deep, steady breaths*, gently gazing towards your nose tip, **dristi: nasagrai**. Allow your face to relax, softening around your eyes and jaw muscles. From Salamba Sarvangasana, move directly into the next asana.

Warning
Do not practise this asana if you have high blood pressure, heart problems, a neck injury, a prolapsed disc, a hernia or glaucoma, or during menstruation (see the moderated posture opposite).

salamba = supported
sarva = entire or whole
anga = limb or body

Using the wall to support the legs in the shoulder stand helps to lift the torso up into vertical alignment. The benefits are the same as in the full pose, but this is a good way to acclimatize oneself to inversions of the body and is wonderfully rejuvenating.

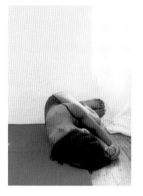

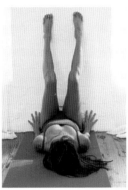

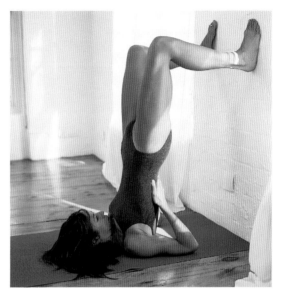

1 Place your yoga mat against the wall and lie on your side, with your knees drawn up, placing your right shoulder and hip along the edge of your mat with your buttocks touching the wall.

2 *Exhale* and roll over on to your back, levelling your buttocks against the wall, and keeping your spine straight. Step your feet up the wall, with your knees bent and your arms by your sides.

3 *Inhale* and press your feet firmly into the wall. Engage uddiyana bandha and raise your pelvis off the floor, lifting up through your back to open your chest up against your chin. Move your whole pelvis up and over your shoulders and draw your elbows in towards one another. Now press your elbows down into the floor and place your palms on your back. *Breathe here for 20–30 full, even breaths*, and then move into the next asana, or release your hands on to the floor and softly roll your back and hips down. Bend your knees and roll on to your right side to come out of this moderated posture.

Benefits of the pose
The action of lifting and pressing the chest up against the chin deepens jalandhara bandha and regulates the thyroid and parathyroid glands situated at the front of the throat. When these glands are balanced, this helps to maintain the health of the digestive, nervous, circulatory and endocrine systems, so ensuring the regeneration of cells, bones and bodily energy.

Deepening the pose
Focus on breathing steadily and slowly. Lift your sternum (breastbone) right up and into your chin to deepen the throat lock, which will stimulate and balance your thyroid gland. If you feel tension building up in your shoulders, softly roll them down into the floor and direct energy from your shoulders through your upper arms and into your elbows. Gently root your elbows down and

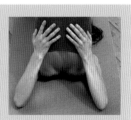

send the energy from your elbows up into your palms to give support into your back and raise your pelvis higher. In this way, we can transform tension into positive energy.

Easing into the pose
If you have health problems (see warning box), instead of raising your pelvis off the floor, simply extend your legs straight up the wall and soften your back, releasing it into the floor with arms outstretched.

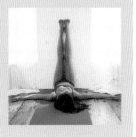

Halāsana | PLOUGH POSTURE

hala = plough

Just as the plough drives through into the darkness of the earth to loosen the soil and uproot the old growth, so, in this asana, the blood is sent through the brain to clear and lighten the mind. It also stretches the arms and back and opens the shoulders.

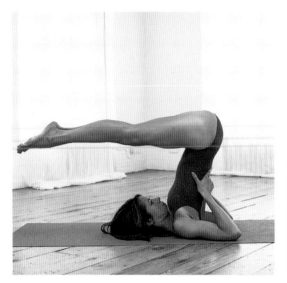
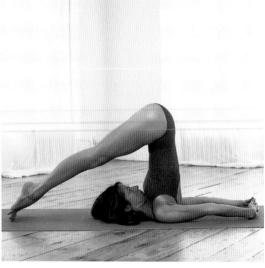

1 After *taking 20–30 breaths* in Salamba Sarvangasana, *exhale* and, while maintaining a strong lift through your abdomen, pubis and buttock bones, hinge your legs out from your hips, lowering your feet towards the floor. Keep your legs lengthening straight and support your back with your hands. Strongly lift your hips and allow the back of your pelvis to move very slightly back towards your hands in order to counter the weight of your legs as they lower down.

2 Continue to *exhale* as you keep lowering your legs with control, bringing your toe tips down on to the floor beyond the top of your head. Raise your buttock bones and pubic bone high, and lengthen through the front of your torso, stretching your front spine long. Release your hands from your back and interlace your fingers deeply, extending your arms straight out behind you. Roll your shoulders down away from your ears, and press your elbows, wrists and little fingers softly into the floor. Draw your collarbones wide, and open your chest up and into your chin to deepen jalandhara bandha. *Take 10–20 full, slow breaths* here before flowing into the next asana. Look towards your nose tip, <u>dristi: **nasagrai**</u>, relaxing your face and softening your jaw.

Easing into the pose

Lowering your feet on to a pre-positioned chair is a soft alternative to Halasana that is exceptionally soothing on your entire nervous system and is particularly beneficial to those who suffer from extreme neck tension and tightness. Bending your knees on to your forehead is another helpful way of easing into the posture of Halasana.

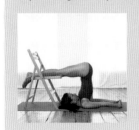
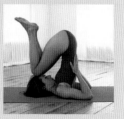

Deepening the pose

Do not stub your toes into the floor. Instead, place the very tops of your toes down and extend your legs long, drawing your kneecaps and thigh muscles up towards your hips, to help the pelvis remain lifted.

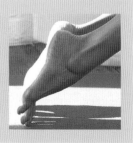

Karṇapīḍāsana | EAR PRESSURE POSTURE

karna = ear
pida = pressure

Drawing the knees on to the ears deepens the stretch through the back, which tones and balances the nervous system. It also closes out external sound, making it possible to listen inwardly to the beat of the heart and the rhythm of breathing.

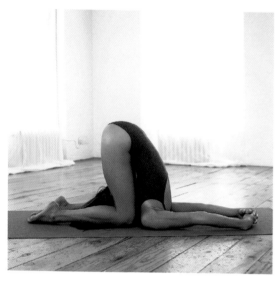

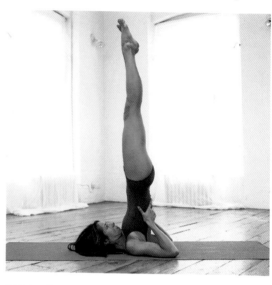

1 From Halasana, *exhale* and bend your knees, allowing them to part. Draw them in towards your ears, while projecting your buttock bones upwards to create length and space in the front of your spine and torso. Softly press your inner knees against your ears and extend your shinbones down on to the floor, stretching through the front of your ankles and feet. Bring your toes and heels together and release mula bandha, while maintaining uddiyana and jalandhara bandha. Lift and open your sternum up against your chin, and extend your arms backwards, gently pressing your elbows and little fingers down into the floor as your hands remain interlaced. *Take 10–20 even breaths*, quietly listening to the sound of your breathing as your knees close out the external sounds, which helps to induce pratyahara (sensory withdrawal). Look towards your nose tip, <u>dristi</u>: nasagrai, and relax behind your eyes.

2 *Inhale*, release your hands from their interlace, and bring your palms on to your back. Draw your knees away from your ears by lengthening your legs straight and together into Halasana. Extend your pelvis upwards and then lift your legs up to return into Salamba Sarvangasana. Re-engage mula bandha, then move directly into the next posture.

Benefits of the pose
This pose intensely stretches the entire length of the spine. It is particularly helpful in alleviating compression around the neck and upper back. Be mindful to distribute your weight evenly through both shoulders to help align the cervical vertebrae.

Easing into the pose
At first, you may find that your shinbones do not reach the floor. Do not try to force them, as this may cause injury to your neck. Instead, tuck your toes under as you draw your knees in, and, as your spine becomes more supple, slowly extend your toes

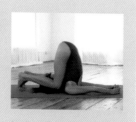

back until your shinbones can gently release down on to the floor.

Deepening the pose
It is also possible to practise this posture by wrapping your arms around the backs of your legs. The weight of your arms will help to send your shinbones further down into the floor.

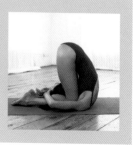

Urdhva Padmāsana | UPWARD LOTUS POSTURE

urdhva = upward
padma = lotus

In this inverted position the posture of Padmasana may be a little easier to achieve, as the legs are made lighter by being lifted. This promotes full mobility and flexibility within the hips and energy circulation through the pelvic region.

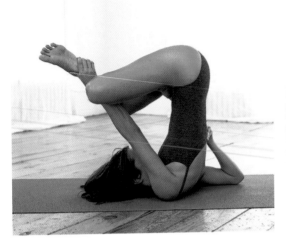

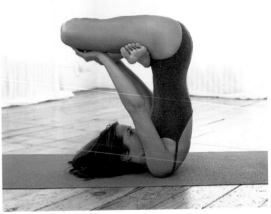

1 While in Salamba Sarvangasana, *exhale*, bend your right knee without dropping your hips, and bring your right foot across to your left upper thigh, as in half lotus. Now draw your left foot across to the top of your right upper thigh to create a full lotus posture in your legs. Use your hands at first to help move your feet across into Padmasana. With practice, you will be able to do this without the help of your hands.

2 Once your legs are securely and comfortably placed in Padmasana, take your hands just under your knees. Lengthen through the front and back of your spine and extend your back straight, with your pelvis balancing directly over and in line with your shoulders. Feel the connection between your palms and your knees and widen your shoulders evenly down into the floor as you straighten your arms, evenly pressing your palms upwards and your knees downwards. This will create a steady balance with your thighs aligned parallel to the floor and your torso and spine completely perpendicular. *Breathe here for 10–20 full breaths*, softly gazing towards your nose tip, **dristi: nasagrai**, then move smoothly into the next asana.

Deepening the pose
This is a wonderful asana to deepen your awareness and engagement of all your bandhas. As your arms straighten and your pelvis lifts, space is created in your front torso, allowing for the complete drawing in of your abdomen into uddiyana bandha. The openness of your chest presses into your chin to strengthen jalandhara bandha. Your pelvic floor and perineum in this

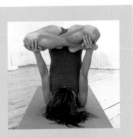

posture have no weight bearing down on them, so the energy of mula bandha can be fully harnessed within. Keep your buttocks level, as this will help you to balance in this pose.

Easing into the pose
If full Padmasana causes knee pain, work into half lotus (Ardha Padmasana), and if half lotus also aggravates your knee joints, cross your ankles and align your feet to float over your buttocks. You may also at first place your hands on your back to help maintain a balance here until you

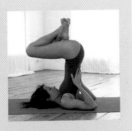

gain greater control to balance with your hands beneath your knees.

Piṇḍāsana | EMBRYO POSTURE

pinda = embryo

In Pindasana the body is drawn into a foetus-like shape, softly curling in upon itself to resemble an embryo within the womb. Further suppleness is developed because the legs remain in Padmasana, creating an inverted forward bend action through the pelvis.

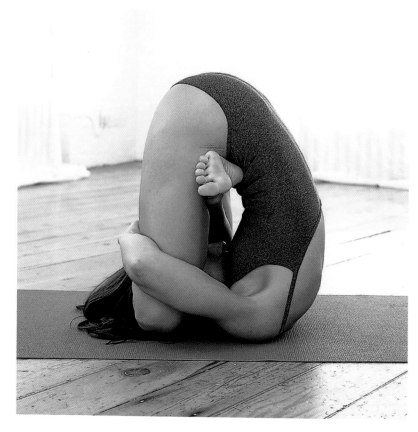

1 Maintaining Padmasana and full engagement of your bandhas, *inhale* and release your hands from your knees, balancing still over your shoulders and neck. With a *slow exhalation*, draw your lotus legs down and in towards your chest, wrapping your arms around your legs to clasp your hands together. Open the backs of your shoulders evenly and release your neck long into the floor to create a broad base on which to balance. Gently move your knees down on either side of your head and feel your body softly curling inwards into an embryo shape, as if resting inside the womb. *Take 10–20 full, even, deep breaths*, looking towards your nose tip, **dristi**: **nasagrai**, and relaxing the space in between your eyebrows to open up your third eye centre. From this asana, move smoothly and directly into the next.

Easing into the pose
As with the previous posture, care must be taken of your knees to prevent injury, so practise this posture with your legs in half lotus, or crossed if knee pain is felt. If, once in lotus, your balance feels unsteady or the stretch through your neck is too extreme at first, place your hands on your back to give your body extra support.

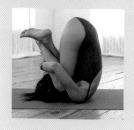
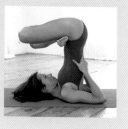

Deepening the pose
As you begin to feel more secure and comfortable in Pindasana, draw your knees closer together and lower your shins or ankles on to your forehead, taking hold of your wrist with your other hand.

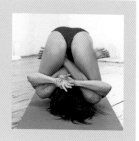

Matsyāsana | FISH POSTURE

matsya = the fish incarnation of Visnu (preserver of the universe and second deity of the Hindu trinity)

This posture provides a complete counter-stretch to the four previous asanas. From the closed curling in of the body into the embryo shape, the back now reverses its position to arch open and stretch through to the front of the throat.

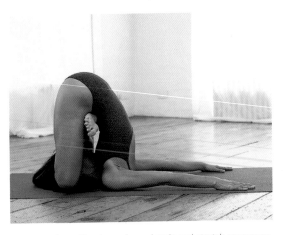

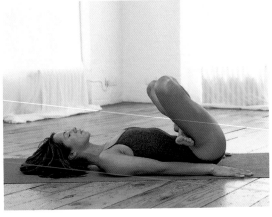

1 *Exhale*, release the clasp of your hands and stretch your arms out behind you, pressing your palms down and extending your fingertips away from your body. Feel your legs securely in the posture of Padmasana (or half lotus or crossed at the ankles, if lotus is not yet possible).

2 Continue to *exhale* and slowly roll down through your spine, sequentially lowering your back vertebra by vertebra on to the floor. Keep the back of your head down and use the pressure of your arms against the ground and the suction of uddiyana bandha to create a fluid roll of your back down on to the floor.

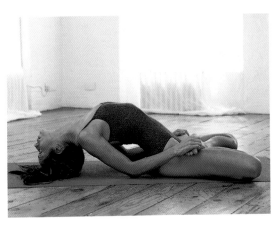

3 As the back of your pelvis touches down, press your knees down on to the floor and arch up through your spine, opening your collarbones wide and lifting your heart skywards. *Complete your exhalation* to release your head back so that the crown of your skull rests on the floor and the front of your throat lengthens long. Take your hands to your feet and roll your elbows in, without them pushing on to the floor. *Breathe here for 10–20 full, deep breaths*, feeling the expansion of your chest and the release of your throat. Softly gaze towards your third eye centre, <u>dristi</u>: **bru madhya**, and relax your facial muscles while drawing your lower jaw up to your upper jaw to stretch your underchin. The next asana, Uttana Padasana, flows on directly from this one.

Easing into the pose
If you practised the last two postures in half lotus or with crossed ankles, you can continue to do so here, but instead of catching hold of your feet, press your palms and forearms down on to the floor by your sides.

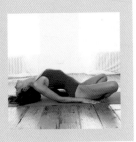

Deepening the pose
Deepen the arch through your back by taking your hands further over your feet and gently pulling on them to raise your chest. As you do so, draw your spine in and up into your body, moving it through into the front of your torso.

Uttāna Pādāsana | EXTENDED FEET POSTURE

uttana = extended or intense stretch
pada = foot or leg

Muscular tone and strength are built through the legs and arms as they stretch up from the floor. The spine arches up, raising and expanding the chest and opening the front of the ribs and lungs to invigorate the heart and enhance deep respiration.

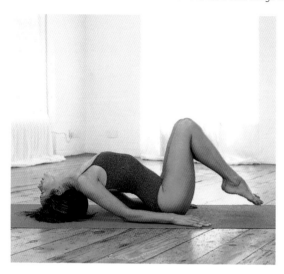

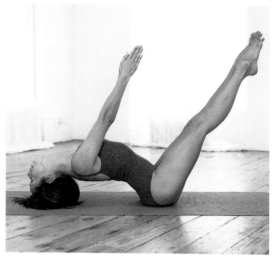

1 From Matsyasana, *inhale*, maintaining the high arch through your spine, and release your feet and legs out of lotus. Draw your inner knees tightly together to activate your inner thighs after their opening in the lotus posture. Stretch long through your shinbones into your feet, not allowing your toes to touch down on to the floor.

2 Continue to *inhale*, and stretch your legs straight, raising them sharply off the floor at a 45–50-degree angle. Extend your arms to follow the same alignment as your legs, and arrow your toe tips and fingertips outwards, lifting through your upper back and pressing your chest high. Draw your kneecaps and thigh muscles up and in towards your hips to stretch your legs fully. Take your focus towards your nose tip, <u>dristi</u>: nasagrai, as you *take 10–20 steady breaths*. *Exhale* as you release your back on to the floor, keeping your legs lifted, and place your palms by the side of your head with your fingertips pointing towards your shoulders.

• With an *inhalation*, roll over your back to complete Chakrasana and move through a **full vinyasa**, but, instead of taking a **jump through** into Dandasana, lower your knees on to the floor to prepare for Sirsasana.

Easing into the pose
If you have back pain or weakness, practise this posture at first by pressing your forearms and hands down on to the floor by the sides of your body. If you have recently suffered a back injury, keep your feet and legs on the floor and press out through your heels to keep your legs active.

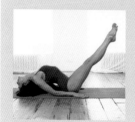
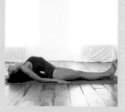

Deepening the pose
Press the back of your waist upwards, tilting your pelvis forwards to balance high up on your sitting bones. Draw your lower abdomen muscles upwards and in towards your navel in order to engage uddiyana bandha deeply. This will give support to your back and the lift of your legs in this asana. Stretch through to your fingertips to energize your arms.

Śīrṣāsana | HEADSTAND POSTURE

sirsa = head

This is the father posture, which harmonizes the effects of Sarvangasana and creates a balance of energies within the body and mind. Here the body stands on the head in an upside down Tadasana, stimulating *sahasrara chakra*, the seat of enlightenment.

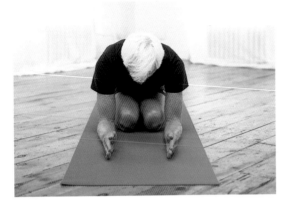

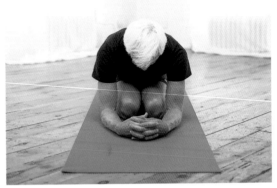

1 From Adho Mukha Svanasana, *inhale* and lower your knees on to the floor. Kneel down with your knees together and bring your hips back over your heels. Place your elbows on either side of your knees, aligned under your shoulders, and stretch your forearms and fingers forwards.

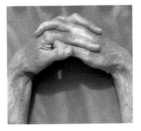

2 Continue to *inhale*, and deeply interlace your fingers, creating a semicircle through the palms (see left). Extend your forearms and elbows down into the floor and draw your shoulders back to open your chest and feel strong through your arms.

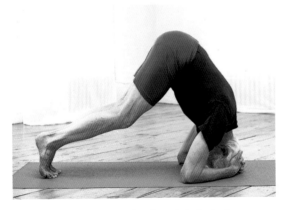

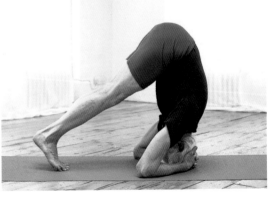

3 As you begin to *exhale*, lengthen through the back of your neck and extend the back of your head into your palms, cupping your head. Lightly place the top of your head on the floor and lift your shoulders up and away from your ears to create space and length in your neck. Engage uddiyana bandha as you tuck your toes under and raise your hips. Press your elbows down and begin to shift your weight evenly on to your forearms and clasped hands to create a tripod-like base for the headstand.

4 Continue to *exhale* as you walk your feet in towards your face and lift your hips further up, drawing them directly over your shoulders. Consciously press down through your arms and slide your shoulder blades upwards to release any compression in your neck.

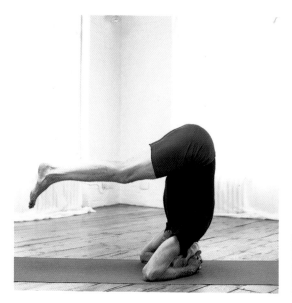

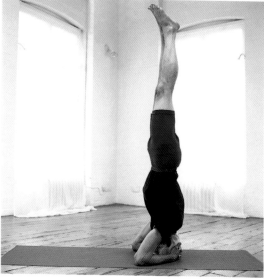

5 When your pelvis is aligned over your shoulders, sway your hips a little further back (this will help you to lever your legs up straight) but keep your toes on the floor for a little longer. Now, *inhale* and deepen your engagement of uddiyana bandha, energize your legs by drawing your kneecaps and thigh muscles up, and then float your feet up off the floor, transferring all your weight on to your arms, and just a little on to your head, and lift your legs to a right angle.

6 Continue to *inhale*, and raise your legs together, stretching them vertically up into the full head balance of Sirsasana. *Take 20–30 steady, deep breaths*, and gaze towards your nose tip, **dristi: nasagrai**, focusing on the support of your forearms and the open evenness through your shoulders. Breathe length into your spine and extend your legs from your hips, as the soles of your feet reach skywards and your elbows and the top of your head root down into earth. From here either go on to step 7 or onto Sirsasana Urdhva Dandasana on page 123.

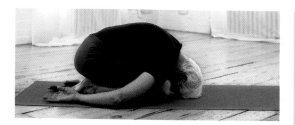

7 Keeping the lift of your pelvis and uddiyana bandha lower your feet to the floor. Bend your knees and sit on your heels into Balasana (child's pose). Lie your forehead onto the floor and take your arms back, with your elbows dropped, and rest here for a full 2 minutes. *Inhale* and place your hands underneath your shoulders, lifting your head and chest up. With your next *exhalation*, **jump back** into Chaturanga Dandasana and move through a **full vinyasa**.

Easing into the pose
If you are still building your confidence with the head balance, you may wish to spring your feet up softly one at a time, gradually working towards springing them up together, until your abdominal strength and confidence develop enough for you to float

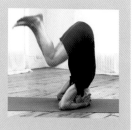

your legs up straight and together.

Deepening the pose
As your strength and confidence build, try moving your elbows and forearms deeper into the floor. Raise your shoulders and lift the top of your head 2.5cm/1in off the ground while maintaining full length through the back of your neck. This is a good test to check that your arms are active and that you are not dropping all your weight into your head and compressing the vertebrae in your neck.

Warning
Do not practise this headstand if you have high blood pressure, heart problems, a neck injury, a prolapsed disc, a hernia or glaucoma, or during menstruation.

Śīrṣāsana Moderations | HEADSTAND POSTURE MODERATIONS

These two moderations, which use a wall for support, assist in the learning of Sirsasana for those who do not feel confident enough to attempt the free-standing form.

As with all asanas, learning from a teacher is always recommended, but for those who are unable to attend classes regularly, these two techniques are helpful.

Moderation A

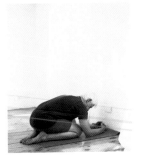 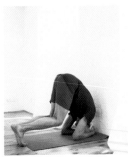 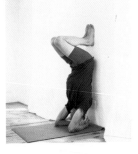 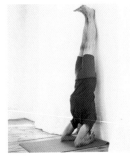

1 Position one end of your folded yoga mat along a wall and kneel down with your knees together. Align your elbows to your outer knees, and deeply interlace your fingers, with your knuckles touching against the wall.

2 Cup the back of your head into your palms and place the top of your head on the mat. Press your forearms down to strengthen the foundations of this posture, and draw your shoulders up. Tuck your toes under, and walk your feet in towards you. Raise your hips, drawing them up and over your shoulders while strongly engaging uddiyana bandha.

3 With an *inhalation*, spring your feet on to the wall.

4 Stretch your legs straight up along the wall. Start with *taking just a few breaths* in the headstand here, and then, with each practice, *add another breath*. As you develop your strength and confidence, begin to move one foot and then the other 2.5cm/1in away from the wall, so you start to find your balance, free-standing on your elbows, forearms and head without the support of the wall. It is very important that you do not become reliant on the wall, it is intended as a temporary aid, not as a permanent fixture of Sirsasana. Rest for a full 2 minutes in Balasana (child's pose).

Moderation B

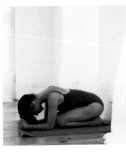 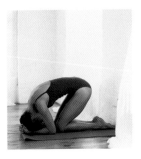 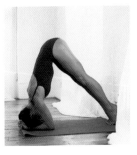 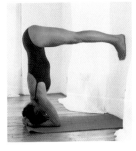

1 Bring yourself into Balasana with the tips of your toes touching the wall, interlacing your fingers ready to cup the back of your head in your palms.

2 Place the top of your head on the mat and extend the back of your head in to your hands. Press your forearms down to secure your base for this posture, then lift your shoulders upwards away from your ears and raise your hips.

3 Tuck your toes under and straighten your legs, keeping your toes still on the floor. Strongly engage uddiyana bandha and lift your hips up.

4 Walk your feet up the wall until your legs are parallel to the ground. Press your hips up and over your shoulders and stretch out through your legs, opening the soles of your feet into the wall. *Breathe steadily here for five breaths*, drawing your shoulders upwards and pressing your elbows down. On the final *exhalation*, walk your feet back down on to the floor and rest in Balasana for a full 2 minutes.

Śīrṣāsana Ūrdhva Daṇḍāsana | HEADSTAND UPWARD STAFF POSTURE

sirsa = head
urdhva = upward
danda = staff, rod or stick

Once a stable headstand has been achieved, this posture, in which the legs are drawn downwards and then sent back up into the full inverted balance, may be tried. This movement stimulates the blood circulation, removing fatigue and tiredness in legs.

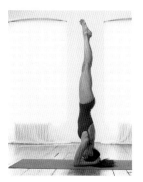 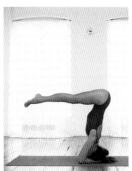

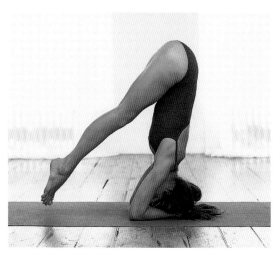

1 After breathing in Sirsasana for *20 breaths*, re-energize your legs by opening the soles of your feet upwards. Refresh the engagement of your bandhas, strongly lift your shoulders up and connect your forearms firmly into the floor to re-establish a sound base for your headstand and the following variation.

2 With a *slow exhalation*, lower your legs to a right angle, strongly projecting your sitting bones up and extending energy down through your arms, while actively sliding your shoulder blades upwards so as not to shorten your neck. Lengthen your legs, feeling the extension through the backs of your thighs, and stretch the backs of your knees straight.

3 Continue to *exhale*, and lower your legs straight down almost to the ground, so that your toe tips hover just 2.5cm/1in or so above the floor. Maintain the lift of uddiyana bandha and the alignment of your pelvis over your shoulders to control the lowering of your legs. Stretch up through your back and open your shoulders, rooting firmly down through your elbows and forearms. With a *full, slow inhalation*, lift your legs up straight again through a right angle and then into the vertical alignment of Sirsasana. Be careful not to tense your shoulders up in the effort to return your legs upright. Uddiyana bandha, along with the *inhalation* and the rooting down into the base created by your arms, needs to be the driving force that floats your legs up.

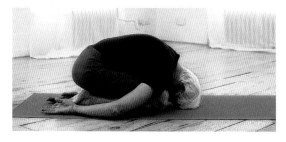

4 Repeat this lowering and lifting of your legs another four times, moving your legs down with an *exhalation* and floating your legs up with an *inhalation*. When you have performed this motion five times in all, lower your feet on to the floor, bend your knees and sit your buttocks back on to your heels. Lower your forehead on to the floor and take your arms back by the sides of your legs, allowing your elbows to drop to the floor. Rest here for a full 2 minutes in Balasana (child's pose).

• *Inhale* and place your hands under your shoulders, lifting your head and chest up. With your next *exhalation*, jump your feet back into Chaturanga Dandasana and move into a **full vinyasa**.

Easing into the pose
Once you feel secure in Sirsasana and can hold it for a full 30 breaths, then you may progress on to this variation. To begin with, move your legs downwards in slow motion so as not to lose control of your balance. As your legs extend forwards, focus on deepening uddiyana bandha and draw your pelvis back very slightly to counter the movement and weight of your legs as they stretch out and down.

Deepening the pose
As you become confident with this variation, you may wish to take five breaths with your legs extending out parallel to the floor before lowering them to let your toe tips hover just 2.5cm/1in or so above the floor.

Baddha Padmāsana | BOUND LOTUS POSTURE

baddha = bound or caught
padma = lotus

In this asana, the arms extend backwards, expanding the chest and lungs and releasing tension and stiffness from the shoulders. The hips and knees are opened, improving flexibility, and the vertebrae of the spine align as the back is drawn straight.

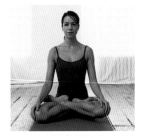 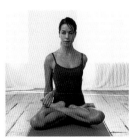

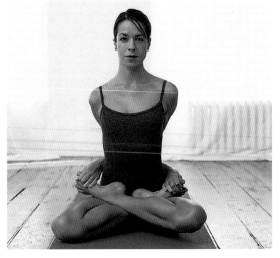

1 From Dandasana, *exhale* and bend your right knee, drawing your right foot up across on to the top of your left upper thigh into half lotus. Continue to *exhale* and bend your left knee, placing your left foot over on to your right upper thigh to come into the full lotus posture of Padmasana. Press your knees in towards one another to ensure your feet are sufficiently placed across your thighs, and fully engage uddiyana bandha. Draw length into your spine and consciously relax your shoulders.

2 With an *inhalation*, softly sweep your left arm back, reaching your hand to your right hip and catching hold of your left big toe with your middle and index fingers.

3 Continue to *inhale* and now extend your right arm behind your back, taking your hand towards your left side to catch hold of your right big toe with your index and middle fingers. *Breathe steadily and fully here for 10–20 breaths,* and gaze softly towards your nose tip, **dristi: nasagrai**. Yield your weight down through your pelvis into the floor, and consciously feel any tension in your body draining down and releasing out on each *exhalation*. As you *inhale* feel energy rebounding up through your back, bringing lightness into your chest and openness across your collarbones. This in turn will help you to release your arms from your shoulders to secure the binding of your hands to your feet. As you complete your *10–20 breaths*, move into Yoga Mudrasana without taking a vinyasa.

Easing into the pose
If you are able to take your legs into full lotus, but not able initially to hold your big toes, use a strap to link your hands to your feet. If pain or strain is felt in your knees, proceed with caution and alternate the full lotus with a half lotus or with Sukhasana (cross-legged), and catch hold of your elbows behind your back.

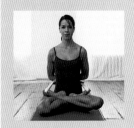 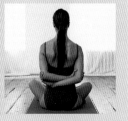

Deepening the pose
As you approach the closing of your practice, the deepening of the yoga postures takes place not only on a physical level but also, more importantly, on a spiritual and mental level. As you breathe here in Baddha Padmasana, cultivate your awareness of sitting in stillness as the internal motion of your breath washes through you.

Yoga Mudrāsana | YOGA SEALING POSTURE

yoga = union
mudra = seal or gesture

Mudras are subtle physical gestures that help to deepen awareness and connect individual energy to the universal energy within. Here, the head bows low to the earth, and the bound hands and feet allow unbroken energy to stream through the body.

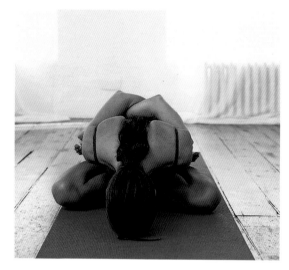

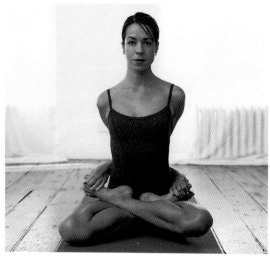

1 From Baddha Padmasana, maintaining an even anchor down through each sitting bone on to the ground, *exhale slowly* and fold your torso forwards, with the top of your head leading your back out and over your feet and legs to bring your face towards the floor. Lengthen long through the front and back of your spine and through into your neck to bring your face down towards the ground. *Take 10–20 deep breaths* here, and focus towards your third eye centre, <u>dristi</u>: **bru madhya**.

2 *Inhale*, drawing your spine upright and straight while keeping hold of your feet. The next posture, Padmasana, follows on directly from here, linked through the *inhalation*.

Easing into the pose
Do not be tempted to roll forwards off your buttocks in an attempt to reach your head all the way down on to the floor, as you will lose your foundation as well as the stretch of this posture. Go only as far as you can with both your sitting bones firmly rooted down into the floor. If you used a strap in Baddha Padmasana to enable you to catch hold of your big toes, continue to work with it here as you extend your torso forwards. If you held your elbows, also continue to do so as you extend your torso forwards.

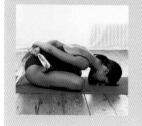

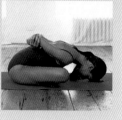

Deepening the pose
Here, again, deepening of the asana is concerned with developing spiritual and mental, as well as physical, awareness. In Yoga Mudrasana, these three elements are intrinsically linked: while practising this asana, deeply engaging your bandhas will increase the benefits of the posture, as the action of the bandhas harnesses the energy of your breath, while the binding gesture of your hands on to your feet seals this harnessed energy within your body, raising your prana to awaken spiritual consciousness. As you breathe in this posture, tune into the flow of your breath washing through your body and mind, removing any blockages as it travels through you.

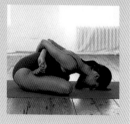

Padmāsana | LOTUS POSTURE

padma = lotus

The lotus posture is often referred to as the royal pose, as energy rises up through the spine to lift the back majestically, directing the flow of prana from the first chakra (*muladhara*) through to the highest chakra of sahasrara at the crown of the head.

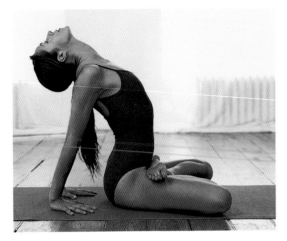

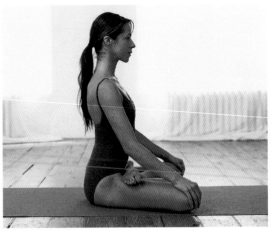

1 Continuing to *inhale*, release your hands from your feet and place your palms face down on to the floor behind your hips with your fingers pointing inwards. Draw up through your lower spine at the same time as pressing down through your sitting bones, hands and knees to send energy up to arch through your back. Lift your chest and open your heart as you release the breath. *Take a full 10–20 breaths*, focusing on expanding your chest with each inhalation, and with each exhalation softly roll your shoulders back and down while relaxing your neck muscles so that your head can gently fall as your heart lifts. Gaze towards your third eye centre, <u>dristi</u>: **bru madhya**.

2 With an *inhalation*, return your head and body to vertical and place your hands to rest on top of your knees. Softly lower your chin and focus to your nose tip, <u>dristi</u>: **nasagrai**. *Take 20–30 full, even breaths here*, yielding weight through into your pelvis to connect to the earth, and feel energy softly rippling up through your spine. Keep your gaze steady and your face relaxed.

• From Padmasana move straight into Tolasana.

Easing into the pose
All the previous asanas have helped you to tune into your body, so if you feel any discomfort or strain in your knees, listen to that warning and place your legs into half lotus, or Sukhasana (cross-legged) instead. If dropping your head back creates tension in your neck, draw your chin down and lift your chest up. Take 20 breaths here, softening the back of the neck while keeping it long.

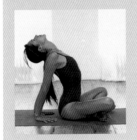

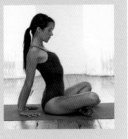

Deepening the pose
Breathe energy and space into your body, mind and heart as you free yourself from physical, mental and emotional restlessness. Allow yourself to drop into the stillness of Padmasana. This is known as practising *kaya sthairyam*, or complete body stillness. When your mind begins to wander and you feel the temptation to fidget, bring your awareness back to the sound and sensation of your breath. Let your pelvis and legs take root, and see your breath streaming up through your spine like a ray of sunlight, bringing illumination and lightness into your mind ... clearing the veils of darkness and obscurations.

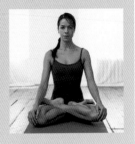

Tolāsana | SCALES POSTURE

tola = a pair of scales

This asana is both demanding and challenging, allowing full appreciation of the relaxation of the closing posture of the sequence, Savasana. The strength of the bandhas is harnessed as Padmasana is raised up through the power of the arms.

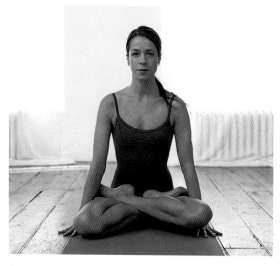

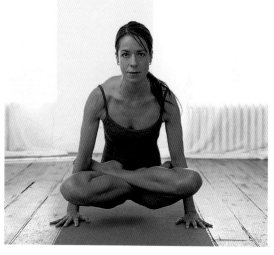

1 *Exhale*, releasing your hands from your knees and placing your palms on the floor by the sides of your hips. Draw your shoulders back and down, maintaining openness across your chest and deeply engaging uddiyana and mula bandha.

2 As you *inhale*, press down through your arms into your palms, and pick your knees up. Now, with full energy, straighten your arms to raise your seat off the floor. *Breathe here for 20–30 full, steady breaths*, focusing towards your nose tip, <u>**dristi: nasagrai**</u>, while maintaining uddiyana bandha. As this is a demanding asana, deepen your ujjayi breathing, feeling energy rising to help float your hips up with each *inhalation*. With each *exhalation* feel energy surging down through your arms and palms to help create a strong connection into the earth.

• *Inhale* and lower yourself back down on to the floor, then release your legs from lotus into Dandasana. Softly flow through your last **full vinyasa** of the practice. The total relaxation of Savasana follows.

Benefits of the pose
This finishing posture helps to cultivate the core strength of your bandhas while strengthening the arms, wrists and hands. As relaxation follows, direct all your energy into mastering this challenging pose.

Easing into the pose
Work this pose with your ankles crossed in Sukhasana if Padmasana is not yet possible. Refer to Lolasana on page 86 to remind yourself of the details.

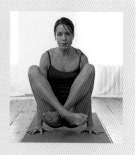

Deepening the pose
Do not rely on the tension of your shoulders to lift your torso and pelvis up. The key to raising your buttocks off the floor is uddiyana bandha. Keep shoulders level and release your shoulder blades down.

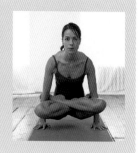

Śavāsana/Mṛtāsana | CORPSE POSTURE

sava and mrta = corpse

True, deep relaxation is the secret to health and happiness. Throughout our lives we accumulate tension, which can inhibit our growth, health, happiness and creativity. To fulfil our potential, therefore, it is necessary to relax fully and drop the tensions away.

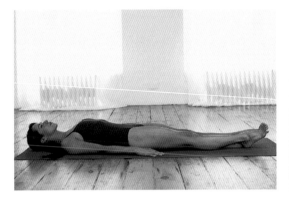

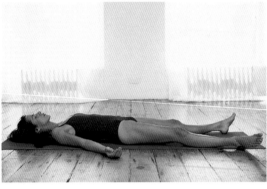

1 From your last vinyasa, jump through into Dandasana and softly roll your back sequentially down on to the floor, to lie in a straight line as you *exhale*.

2 Move your feet apart a little wider than your hips. Allow your breath to flow naturally and release your arms out to the sides of your body, turning your palms to face upwards. With a *deep exhalation*, sink your whole body into the ground, feeling the ground beneath you softening to receive the weight and shape of your body. As you lie here, slowly rotate your consciousness through your entire body, relaxing and allowing each and every part in turn to melt as it makes contact with the ground.

Deepening the pose
Savasana is one of the most important of all postures, and the way in which to deepen this asana is to carry it into the context of our everyday lives, practising not to hold on, allowing ourselves truly to let go in our body, mind and heart. In this way we can open up our lives to newness.

Benefits of the pose
The relaxation induced by Savasana allows your body and mind to absorb the harmonizing benefits and energy that have been generated through all the postures that have come before this point of your practice.

Breath by breath in Savasana, let tension flow out from your skin, muscles, organs, bones and cells, consciously relaxing your mind by consciously relaxing your body.

The series has cleansed, unblocked and released your body and mind from stagnant energy, tensions and toxins. Now the purified body may rest unburdened in this clear open space.

Listen within to the sound of your breath, the sensation of your body, the consciousness of your mind and the awareness of your heart.

As you relax in Savasana, the parasympathetic (relaxatory) and sympathetic (excitatory) nervous systems balance, inducing a state of yogic sleep (*yoganidra*). This enables you to discover an internal sanctuary of deep relaxation with inner awareness. This is a form of pratyahara, which leads the way to a higher realization.

Through the sensory withdrawal of yoganidra, your breath flows, saturating your body with the vital life energy of prana. This brings healing and rejuvenation into your entire being on every level – from cellular to intellectual – and allows the release of tensions, dramas, old habits and patterns (*samskaras*) from your life. This posture of the corpse drops and surrenders your bones into the ground.

In yogic thought, death is seen not as the end but rather as the route to rebirth. It is the stillness of the sea that pours in between the rising ripples of two waves.

...to make an end is to make a beginning...
the end is where we start from...
with the drawing of this love and the voice of this call
we shall not cease from exploration
and the end of all our exploring
will be to arrive where we started
and know that place for the first time.

T. S. Eliot

Once you are in Savasana

Starting at your head, move your awareness through your body, relaxing and softening each area as you go.

- Feel your skull heavy on the floor, relaxing all your neck muscles and softening your jaw.
- Feel your shoulders falling into the ground, and your elbows, wrists and hands heavy.
- Soften your chest and feel your ribs and stomach fall and rise with each breath.
- Relax your buttocks, feeling your thighs heavily releasing down and out from your hips.
- Soften your knees, relaxing all the way through to your calves and shins.
- Relax in your ankles, feeling your heels sinking into the floor as your toes relax.

- Return your awareness to your head and soften the skin over your face, relaxing your lips.
- Soften your cheeks and melt your eyes into the pools of their sockets.
- Relax the space in between your eyebrows and feel your brain softening gently within its skull.
- Keep warm and spread a blanket over you so that you can spend time here totally relaxing.
- Breathe, soften and release, sinking the landscape of your body into the floor. Feel tension melting away, breath by breath.
- As you lie here, free your body from the perpetual motion of doing and your mind from the wandering of listless thoughts, allowing yourself to rest in stillness, between the waves of your breath.

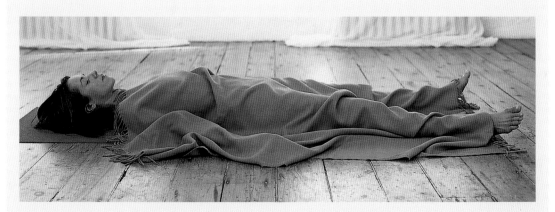

Variations to the pose

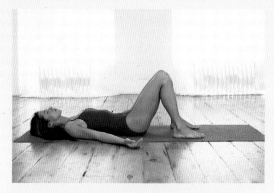

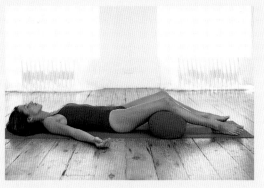

If your lower back feels tense and tends to arch off the floor, rest in Savasana with your knees bent and softly release the small of your back down into the ground with each exhalation.

Alternatively, you may also wish to place cushions or a bolster under your knees, releasing the pressure on your lower back.

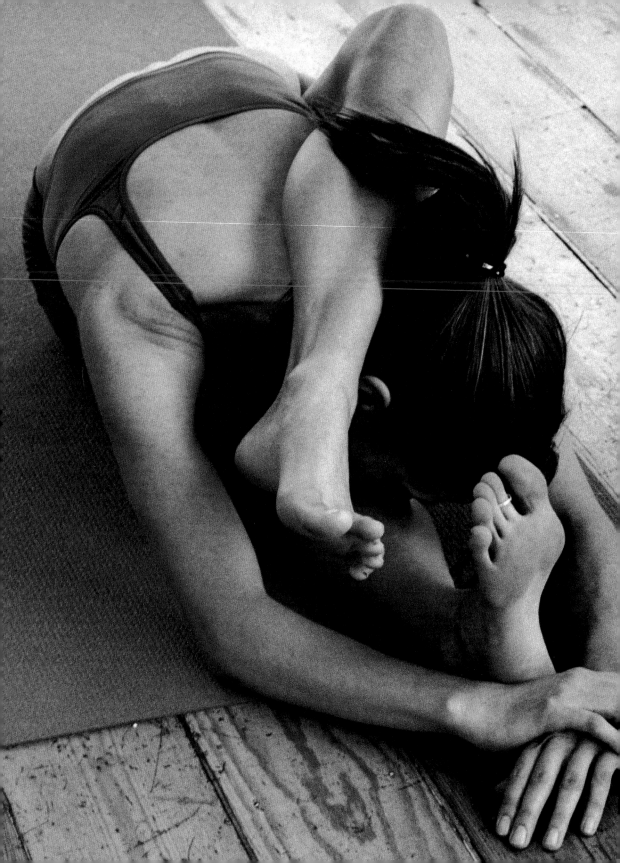

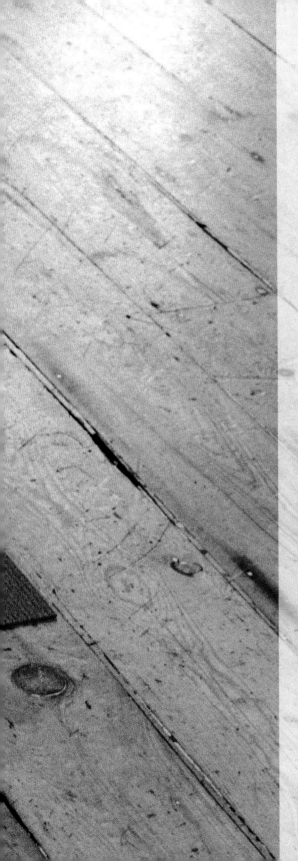

Abridged Sequences

The following sequences are designed for those occasions when we simply do not have enough hours in the day to practise the full primary series. Even though your time may be limited, do not be tempted to race through these postures. Take at least five full, deep breaths in each asana and practise the postures on both the right and left sides to work the body evenly.

Practising yoga a little and often is far more beneficial and balanced than doing a two-hour session once or every other week. Regular practice is the key, even if you only have 15 minutes to do it. It is better to practise fewer postures slowly and calmly than to practice more postures in rush and hurry. Rather than feeling stressed about practice, do what you can and enjoy your time practising the postures.

15-minute Practice

The 15-minute sequence is composed entirely of moderated postures for those who are tired or recovering from injury, or who need a gentle route into the primary series. This gentle sequence of postures has a soothing effect on the nervous system, so it is ideal to practise after a hard day's work or even later on in the evening to help induce sleep. Start by practising Surya Namaskara A twice, and Surya Namaskara B twice, stepping rather than jumping back into Chaturanga Dandasana. Take a minimum of five breaths in each of the standing and sitting postures and be sure to practise the asanas on the both the right and the left side. Props may be used to ease into the postures.

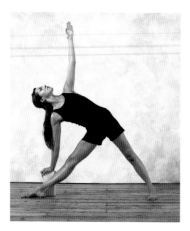

1 Utthita Trikonasana Extended triangle posture moderated p52

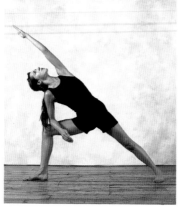

2 Utthita Parsvakonasana Extended lateral angle posture moderated p54

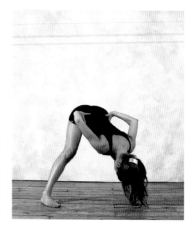

3 Prasarita Padottanasana B Expanded leg stretch posture moderated p57

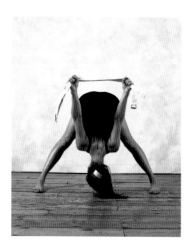

4 Prasarita Padottanasana C Expanded leg stretch posture moderated p58

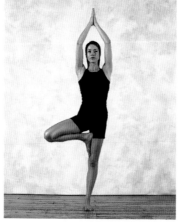

5 Ardha Baddha Padmottanasana Half bound lotus intense stretch posture moderated/ Tree pose p64

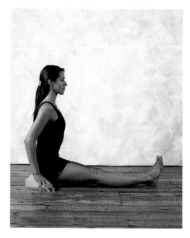

6 Dandasana Staff Posture moderated p72

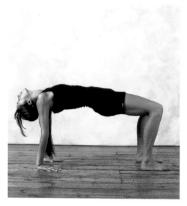

7 Purvottanasana Stretch of the East posture moderated p76

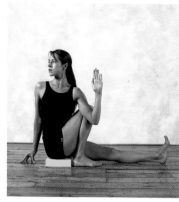

8 Marichyasana C Posture C dedicated to the great sage marichi moderated p84

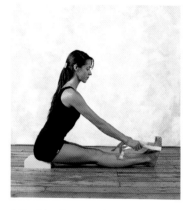

9 Paschimottanasana Intense stretch of the West posture moderated p72

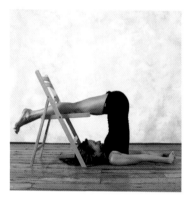

10 Halasana Plough posture moderated p114

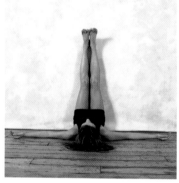

11 Salamba Sarvangasana Supported whole body posture moderation p113

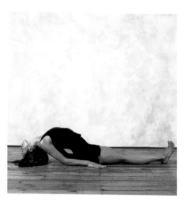

12 Matsyasana moderated Fish posture with legs out-stretched p119

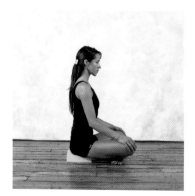

13 Sukhasana Easy happy posture moderated p26

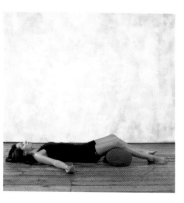

14 Savasana Corpse posture moderated p129

30-minute Practice

This 30-minute yoga session includes the basic key postures and so provides a good intermediatory practice in order to begin to build the strength, stamina and concentration needed for the full series. It is an energizing sequence, so you may wish to make some time for this practice in the morning, as it is a great way to start your day. It will awaken your body and clear your mind of sleepiness while boosting your metabolism. In the mornings, the body may not feel as supple as it does later on in the day, but a couple of extra breaths in each asana will help you to ease a little deeper into the postures without straining. Start this sequence by flowing through Surya Namaskara A three times, and through Surya Namaskara B twice. If you are pressed for time, practise half rather than full vinyasas between asanas.

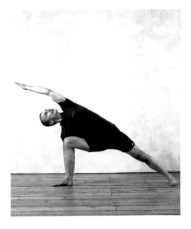

1 Padangusthasana Foot big toe posture p50

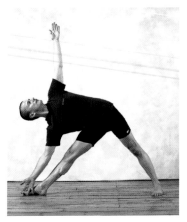

2 Utthita Trikonasana Extended triangle posture p52

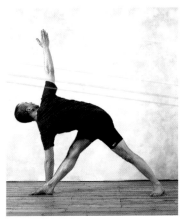

3 Parivrtta Trikonasana Revolved triangle posture p53

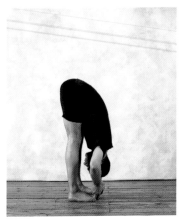

4 Utthita Parsvakonasana Extended lateral angle posture p54

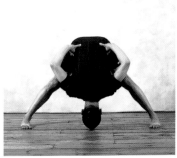

5 Prasarita Padottanasana B Expanded leg stretch posture B p57

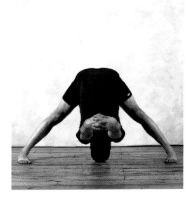

6 Prasarita Padottanasana C Expanded leg stretch posture C p58

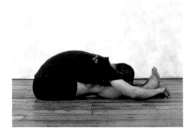

7 Paschimottanasana D Intense stretch of the West posture D p73

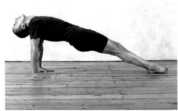

8 Purvottasana Stretch of the East p76

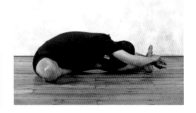

9 Janu Sirsasana A Knee head posture A p79

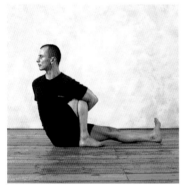

10 Marichyasana C Posture C dedicated to the great sage Marichi p84

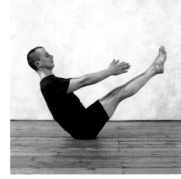

11 Navasana Boat posture p86

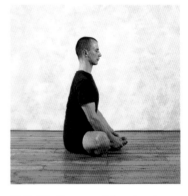

12 Baddha Konasana A Bound angle posture A p94

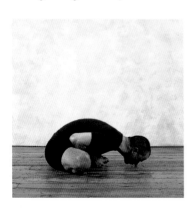

13 Baddha Konasana B Bound angle posture B p94

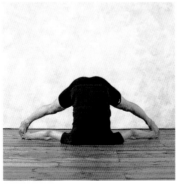

14 Supta Konasana A Sleeping angle posture A p97

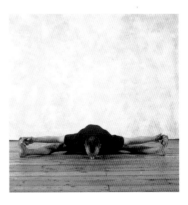

15 Supta Konasana B Sleeping angle posture B p98

▷

30-minute practice continued

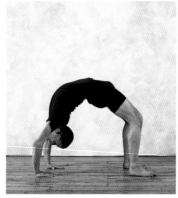

16 Urdhva Dhanurasana Upward bow posture p106

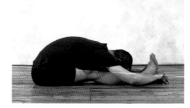

17 Paschimottanasana D Stretch of the West posture D p73

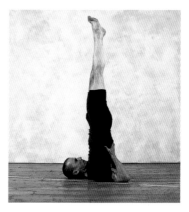

18 Salamba Sarvangasana Supported whole body posture p112

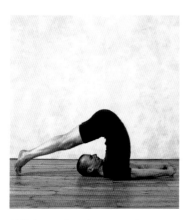

19 Halasana Plough posture p114

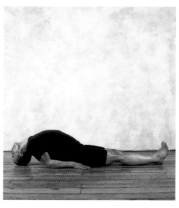

20 Matsyasana moderated Fish posture with legs out-stretched p119

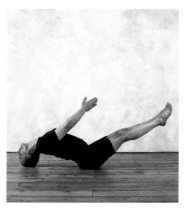

21 Uttana Padasana Extended feet posture p119

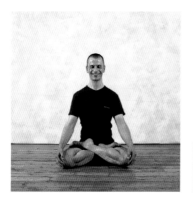

22 Padmasana Lotus posture p126

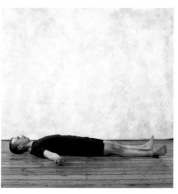

23 Savasana Corpse posture p128

45-minute Practice

This 45-minute routine creates a dynamic practice and is a definite step up from the previous 30-minute sequence. Before moving on to this sequence, therefore, make sure you are familiar with all the postures from the previous one, as the key asanas are now incorporated and developed with the inclusion of some of the more challenging postures.

The full finishing series of asanas included at the end will calm the mind and bodily system from the practice. This sequence may be practised at any time of the day, although it is generally considered to be most beneficial to practise in the morning at sunrise or in the evening at sunset.

Begin this 45-minute session by practising Surya Namaskara A and B three times each. As previously, replace full vinyasas with half vinyasas in between each asana if short of time. Practise mindful breathing throughout all of your postures, and five breaths on each side of a pose.

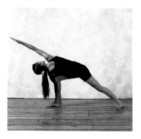

1 Pada Hastasana Foot hand posture p51

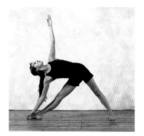

2 Utthita Trikonasana Extended triangle posture p52

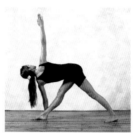

3 Parivrtta Trikonasana Revolved triangle posture p53

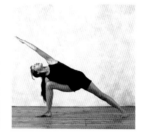

4 Utthita Parsvakonasana Extended lateral angle p54

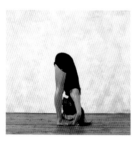

5 Parivrtta Parsvakonasana Revolved lateral angle p55

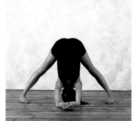

6 Prasarita Padottanasana C Expanded leg stretch C p58

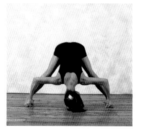

7 Prasarita Padottanasana D Expanded leg stretch D p59

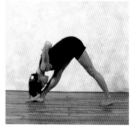

8 Parsvottanasana Side intense stretch posture p60

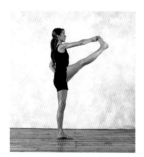

9 Utthita Hasta Padangusthasana Extended hand big toe posture p61

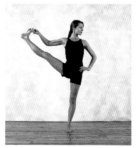

10 Utthita Parsvasahita Extended side posture p62

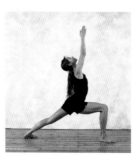

11 Virabhadrasana I Warrior posture I p66

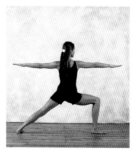

12 Virabhadrasana II Warrior posture II p67

▷

45-minute practice continued

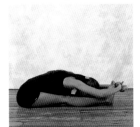

13 Paschimottanasana D
Stretch of the West D p73

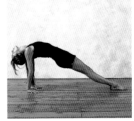

14 Purvottanasana Stretch
of the East posture p76

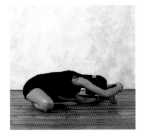

15 Janu Sirsasana B
Knee head posture B p80

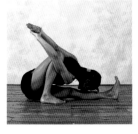

16 Marichyasana A
Sage Marichi A posture p82

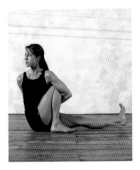

17 Marichyasana C
Sage Marichi posture C p84

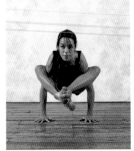

18 Bhujapidasana
Arm pressure posture p87

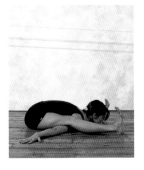

19 Kurmasana Tortoise
posture p89

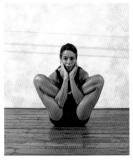

20 Garbha Pindasana A
Womb embryo posture A p92

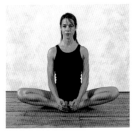

21 Baddha Konasana A
Bound angle posture A p94

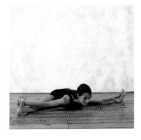

22 Upavista Konasana A
Seated angle posture A p95

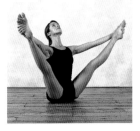

23 Upavista Konasana B
Seated angle posture B p96

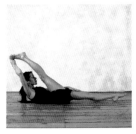

24 Supta Padangusthasana
Sleeping foot big toe p99

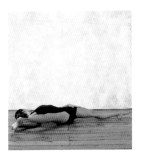

25 Supta Parsvasahita A
Sleeping side posture A p100

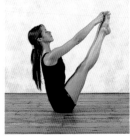

26 Ubhaya Padangusthasana
Both feet big toe posture B p103

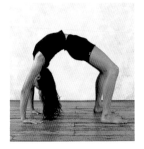

27 Urdhva Dhanurasana
Upward bow posture p106

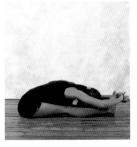

28 Paschimottanasana D
Stretch of the West D p73

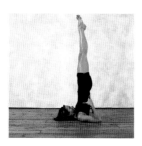

29 Salamba Sarvangasana
Supported body posture p112

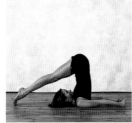

30 Halasana Plough
posture p114

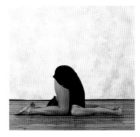

31 Karnapidasana Ear
pressure posture p115

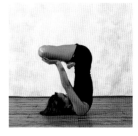

32 Urdhva Padmasana
Upward lotus posture p116

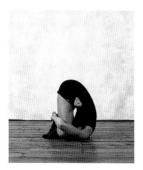

33 Pindasana Embryo
posture p117

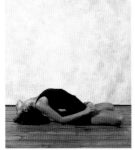

34 Matsyasana Fish
posture p118

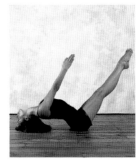

35 Uttana Padasana
Extended feet posture p119

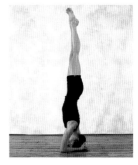

36 Sirsasana Headstand
posture p120

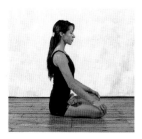

37 Padmasana Lotus
posture p126

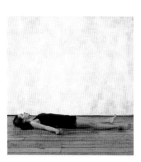

38 Savasana Corpse
posture p128

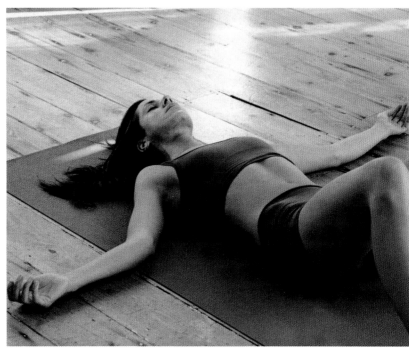

Sanskrit Pronunciation

The yoga asanas are named in Sanskrit, the original language of yoga and ancient India, which reveals the inner meaning of each posture and describe their source of inspiration – for instance, warriors (Virabhadrasana – hero virabhadra), seers and sages (Marichyasana – the sage Marichi), animals (Kurmasana – tortoise), birds (bakasana), plants (Padmasana – lotus), structures (halasana – plough).

Sanskrit is the mother language and is considered to be the oldest language in the world. The Vedas, Upanisads and much of Buddhist literature is written in Sanskrit, which has attracted language and religious scholars worldwide. It is scientific and systematic in its grammatical approach and has been sited as "the only unambiguous language on the planet" by NASA.

There is much debate over the antiquity of the Sanskrit language; it is the precursor of Greek and Latin and is known to date back to at least 1800BC, many experts believe 6000BC to be a more accurate calculation. Over this vast period of time Sanskrit has remained true to its original form, so that someone speaking it today would be perfectly understood by someone who spoke the language 2,000 years ago.

The actual translation of Sanskrit means the "perfected language", whilst its alphabet is called *devanagiri*, which means "cities of gods". The pronunciation of its vowels and consonants is centred around the purity of sound and rhythm, and it is understood that Sanskrit evolved as a result of humans expressing the search and discovery of their divine nature.

The ancient language of Sanskrit is used in the naming of the postures, breathing practices and philosophical concepts of yoga, and learning the original names and their true translations will help to deepen your understanding of the asanas and philosophy of yoga.

The first syllable is always emphasized and this emphasis is lengthened when a diacritic is placed above the vowel.

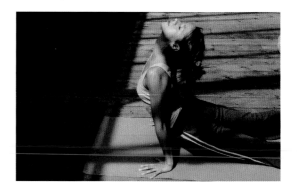

Thus: ā is pronounced ar
        ī is pronounced ee
        ū is pronounced oo

ṭ, ṭh, ḍ, ḍh and ṇ are all spoken with the tongue curled back and hitting the upper palate while the same letters without the dots are pronounced with the tip of the tongue touching the back of the front teeth.

ḥ indicates that the repetition of the preceding vowel needs to be pronounced. For example aḥ becomes aha; uḥ becomes uhu.

    ṅ comes before g or k
    ñ comes before c or j
    ṁ precedes a consonant
    jñ is pronounced gnya
    ṛ is spoken as ri or ru
    ś and ṣ are both pronounced as ssh. For example śīrṣāsana
      (headstand) is pronounced sshirsshasana and
      pārśvakoṇāsana is pronounced parsshvakonasana.

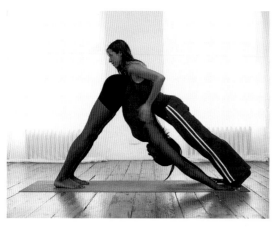

FURTHER READING

Light on Yoga, B.K.S. Iyengar
Yoga Mala, Sri K. Pattabhi Jois
Hatha Yoga: The Hidden Language, Swami Sivananda Radha
The Shambhala Encyclopedia of Yoga, Georg Feuerstein
Asana Pranayama Mudra Bandha, Swami Satyananda Saraswati
Ashtanga Yoga, Lino Miele
Heart of Yoga, Developing a Personal Practice, T.K.V. Desikachar
*A Systematic Course in The Ancient Tantric Techniques of Yoga and
  Kriya*, Swami Satyananda Saraswati
When Things Fall Apart: Heart Advice for Difficult Times, Pema Chödrön
Old Path, White Clouds: Walking in the Footsteps of the Buddha,
  Thich Nhat Hanh
Chakras: Energy Centres of Transformation, Harish Johari

RETREATS
Jean Hall
www.yogajeannie.com
Astanga Yoga Research Centre
www.sharathyogacentre.com
Free Spirit Travel
www.freespirityoga.co.uk

UNITED KINGDOM
Jean Hall
www.instagram.com/yogajeannie
www.movementformodernlife.com/yogateacher/jeanhall

Yogahome
14 Allen Road
London, N16 8SP
Tel. 020 7249 2425
www.yogahome.co.uk

Battersea Yoga
2 Kite Yard
Cambridge Road
London SW11 4TA
info@batterseayoga.com
www.batterseayoga.com

Triyoga
57 Jamestown Road
London, NW1 7DB
Also centres in Chelsea, Ealing, Shoreditch and Soho, London
Tel. 020 7483 3344
www.triyoga.co.uk

Sivananda Yoga Vedanta Centre
51 Felsham Road
London SW15 1AZ
Tel. 020 8780 0160
www.sivanandalondon.org

Satyananda Yoga Centre
70 Thurleigh Road

London SW12 8UD
Tel. 020 8673 4869
www.syclondon.com

Iyengar Yoga Institute
223A Randolph Avenue
Maida Vale
London W9 1NL
Tel. 020 7624 3080
www.iymv.org

The British Wheel of Yoga
25 Jermyn Street
Sleaford
Lincolnshire NG34 7RU
Tel. 01529 306 851
office@bwy.org.uk
www.bwy.org.uk

The Life Centre
15 Edge Street
London W8 7PN
Tel. 020 7221 4602
info@thelifecentre.com
www.thelifecentre.com

The Yoga Shala
Third Floor
1 Chestnut Road
London SE27 9EZ
Tel. 020 8670 7711
www.theshalahlondon.com

USA
The Ashtanga Yoga Center
412 North Coast Hwy
101 Encinitas CA 92024
Tel. 760-566-6824
www.ashtangayogacenter.com

Manju Jois
(son of Sri K. Pattabhi Jois)
www.manjujois.com

Ashtanga Yoga Studio
5117 Macarthur Blvd N.W.
Washington,
D.C. 20016

Tel. (202) 556-0371
info@aysdc.com
www.aysdc.com

Ashtanga Yoga Shala
638 E6th Street
New York, NY 10009
www.ashtangayoga.nyc

The Ashtanga Yoga School
1412 12th Avenue
Seattle, WA 98122
Tel. 206-261-1711
www.yogaspirals.com

Ashtanga Yoga Santa Barbara
324E State Street
Santa Barbara, CA 93101
Tel. 805 965 7175
www.ashtangasantabarbara.com

AUSTRALIA
Astanga Yoga Centre of Melbourne
110-112 Argyle St
Fitroy VC 3065
Tel. 61 421 799 365
www.astangamelbourne.com.au

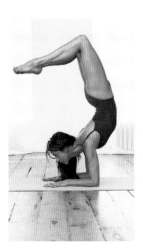

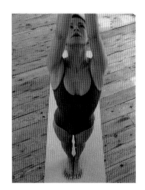

Ashtanga Yoga Moves
30 Alma Street
Paddington 2021 NSW
Tel. 61 2936 07602
www.yogamoves.com.au

Ashtanga Yoga Shala
10 Moreton Street
Paddington 4064
Queensland
Tel. 61 3345 1122
www.ashtangayogashala.com.au

Studio Cirq
6 Laser Drive
Rowville 3178
Tel. 03 9753 4411
www.studiocirq.com.au

NEW ZEALAND
Te Aro Astanga Yoga
116 Cuba Street
Wellington, 6011
Tel. 21 0272 2362
info@astanga.co.nz
www.astanga.co.nz

The Yoga Academy
190 Federal Street
Central City
Auckland 1001
Tel. 64 9 357 0750
yoga@yoga.co.nz
www.yoga.co.nz

Index

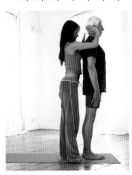

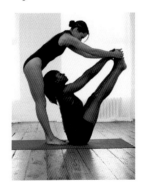

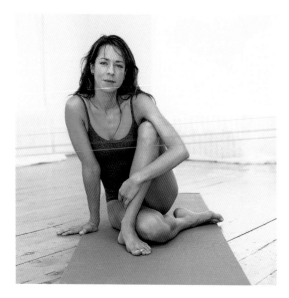

ABOUT THE AUTHOR Jean Hall has spent much of her life exploring bodywork disciplines, travelling, and practising yoga. She discovered yoga whilst training as a dancer. It soon then became an integral part of her life, developing alongside her career as a contemporary performer and, perhaps more importantly, alongside her own personal learning and growth.

She originally qualified as an Iyengar yoga teacher in 1995, and since then has continued to study different forms of yoga, movement and spiritual practices with many great teachers from diverse backgrounds. Of particular influence has been Pema Chödrön, Gill Clarke and Body Mind Centering.

Through collaborating with other teachers and artists who share a flame for the expressive body, Jean continues to teach open yoga classes, workshops, retreats and courses in London, internationally and online.

She is co-founder of both the Daoist Flow Yoga Teacher Training and Triyoga's Advanced Teacher Training programmes.

Jean holds an MA in Performing Arts and is a qualified Senior Yoga Teacher with Yoga Alliance Professionals UK, and an Experienced Registered Yoga Teacher (E-RYT-500) with Yoga Alliance US.

This edition is published by Lorenz Books
an imprint of Anness Publishing Ltd
info@anness.com
www.annesspublishing.com

© Anness Publishing Ltd 2021

A CIP catalogue record for this book is available from the British Library.

Publisher: Joanna Lorenz
Editorial Director: Helen Sudell
Project Editor: Katy Bevan
Designer: Lisa Tai
Cover Designer: Nigel Partridge
Photography: Clare Park
Production Controller: Ben Worley
Models: Jean Hall, Sandra Powell,
   Steven Haines and Grant Jones

PUBLISHER'S ACKNOWLEDGEMENTS

Thanks for the loan of props to Paul Walker at Yoga Matters, suppliers of yoga mats, props and clothing. 32 Clarendon Road, London N8 ODJ, 020 8888 8588 fax 020 8888 0623 www.yogamatters.co.uk (www.yogapropshop.com) Thank you to Stuart Mackay at Beyond Hope for supplying the prAna clothing. Contact www.prana.com for stockists.
The Art Archive/The British Library p13 bl and p27 tr. Nathan Rabe p10 bl. Penny Brown p27b, p29. Shutterstock p13br, 16, 27t.
T. S. Eliot's Little Gidding quoted courtesy of Faber and Faber Ltd.

AUTHOR'S ACKNOWLEDGEMENTS

With thanks to my family, friends and students for their support and kindness. My deepest respect and gratitude to the past and present teachers of the yoga tradition who share and pass on their insight, wisdom and knowledge, and in particular my own teacher Gill Clarke who continues to be a constant source of inspiration, Tessa Bilder for illuminating the inner journey, Anya Evans for installing the value of discipline. Thanks to our models, Steve, Sandra, Grant. Clare Park and Matthew for photography, styling and discretion.